Quick Hits for Pediatric Emergency Medicine

Cristina M. Zeretzke-Bien • Tricia B. Swan

Editors

Quick Hits for Pediatric Emergency Medicine

Second Edition

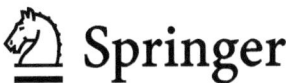 Springer

Editors
Cristina M. Zeretzke-Bien
Division of Pediatric Emergency Medicine
University of Florida
Gainesville, FL, USA

Tricia B. Swan
Division of Pediatric Emergency Medicine
University of Florida
Gainesville, FL, USA

ISBN 978-3-031-32649-3   ISBN 978-3-031-32650-9   (eBook)
https://doi.org/10.1007/978-3-031-32650-9

This Springer imprint is published by the registered company Springer Nature Switzerland AG
The registered company address is: Gewerbestrasse 11, 6330 Cham, Switzerland

Foreword

A lot has changed since I began my pediatric emergency medicine (PEM) fellowship program in 1989. It was an exciting time as there were only about 15 PEM fellowship programs in the country, pediatric advanced life support and resuscitation courses were beginning, the Emergency Medical Services (EMS) for Children Program was rapidly developing, the concept of pediatric weight and length-based medication dosing and equipment was introduced, and pediatric trauma systems of care were rapidly evolving. I was fortunate to train under the guidance of Drs. Robert Luten and Joseph J. Tepas, pioneers and champions in pediatric emergency and trauma care. Pediatric Emergency Medicine became an approved subspecialty in 1991 followed by development of the Pediatric Emergency Care Research Network (PECARN), the National Pediatric Readiness Project, and the rapid growth of the specialties of PEM, EMS, pediatric critical care, and trauma. Fast forward to 2023, there are now over 85 PEM fellowship programs in the US and Canada and a rapid growth of satellite or off-site emergency departments (EDs). Despite the US having almost 200 children's hospitals, the majority of children receive initial emergency care in community or nonchildren's EDs. This book is essential for emergency care providers to be prepared for a critically ill or injured child. All EDs and EMS agencies need a level of pediatric readiness, especially during an unexpected disaster situation. This is especially true for infants as they have a higher presentation rate than other pediatric emergency patients and present unique treatment challenges. Emergency care professionals must be able to rapidly transition from an adult with a stroke to an unexpected newborn delivery to a child with a seizure! This book is great reference for quick pediatric tips, algorithms, and pearls when time is of the essence and you want to care for a pediatric emergency patient as you would compassionately and expertly care for your own child, neighbor, or relative. The book has been edited by two wonderful pediatric emergency physicians, mothers, and educators that I was fortunate to train and mentor. They are now "paying it forward" for others. Children do not come with a manual or phone app so it is important to have key resources to help you navigate their world and decrease your stress level. The greatest honor is to care for another person's child.

Phyllis L. Hendry
Department of Emergency Medicine, University of
Florida College of Medicine/Jacksonville,
Jacksonville, FL, USA

Contents

Chapter 1
Airway: Pediatric Anatomy, Infants, and Children

Cristina M. Zeretzke-Bien

Abstract Kids are not small adults, and their airways are different. Here we have an excellent image of the differences with pediatric airway anatomy and the classic seven Ps for intubation. This is a must-have quick reference for the pediatric airway.

Before You Intubate: What You Need to Know

Kids are not small adults, and their airways are different.

1. Pediatric airway anatomy: *see* Fig. 1.1
2. Obligate nasal breathers
3. Adenoidal hypertrophy
4. Large tongue
5. Large occiput
6. Larynx and trachea are funnel shaped.
7. Vocal cords slant anteriorly.
8. Larynx located higher in the neck (at C4 vs. C6 in adults)
9. Narrowest part of the pediatric airway is at cricoid cartilage (until age 5). In adults, the narrowest part is at the glottis opening.
10. Glottis different locations:

    (a) Premature babies at C3
    (b) Newborns C3–C4
    (c) Adults C5

C. M. Zeretzke-Bien (✉)
Division of Pediatric Emergency Medicine, University of Florida, Gainesville, FL, USA
e-mail: zeretzke@ufl.edu

© The Author(s), under exclusive license to Springer Nature
Switzerland AG 2023
C. M. Zeretzke-Bien, T. B. Swan (eds.), *Quick Hits for Pediatric Emergency Medicine*, https://doi.org/10.1007/978-3-031-32650-9_1

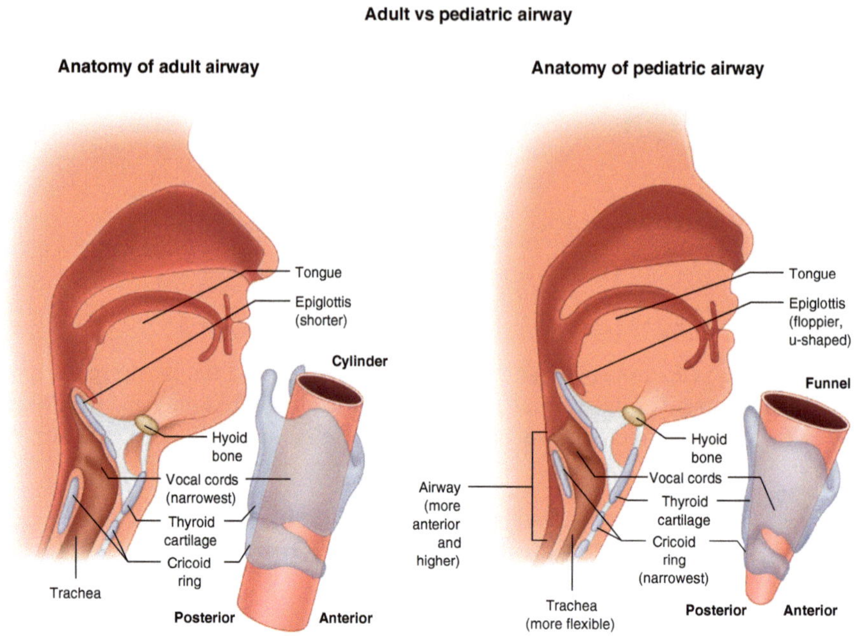

Adult vs pediatric airway

Anatomy of adult airway   **Anatomy of pediatric airway**

Fig. 1.1 Pediatric airway differences: adults and pediatric

Lung Physiology

- Fewer and smaller alveoli (surface area reaches an adult around age 8)
- Channels for collateral ventilation: Pores of Kohn and channels of Lambert

  – Important with atelectasis and alveolar hypoventilation

Lung Mechanics

- Ribs are more horizontal (hard to recruit accessory muscles).
- Thoracic skeleton is cartilaginous and very compliant (important with tidal volume).
- Accessory respiratory muscles: (muscle fibers are slow twitch) more susceptible to fatigue
- Reduced FRC (functional residual capacity)
- Poiseuille's law: Airway resistance is inversely proportional to the fourth power of the radius of the airway (edema, obstruction, secretions).

- Cellular oxygenation: Resting oxygen consumption in the newborn twice in an adult

  - (6 ml/kg/min vs. 3 ml/kg/min)

Tips for Intubation

Seven Ps.

7 P's
  - **P**repare = equipment
  - **P**retreat = drugs
  - **P**osition = sniffing position (if possible)
  - **P**reoxygenate= 100 % pulse ox (consider apneic oxygenation during direct laryngoscopy) [1]
  - **P**aralyze = drugs
  - **P**lacement = tube through cords
  - **P**osition = confirm with ETC02 then CXR

1.Weingart, S and Levitan, R. Preoxygenationand prevention of desaturation during emergency airway management. Ann Emerg Med. 2012 Mar; 59(3):165–175

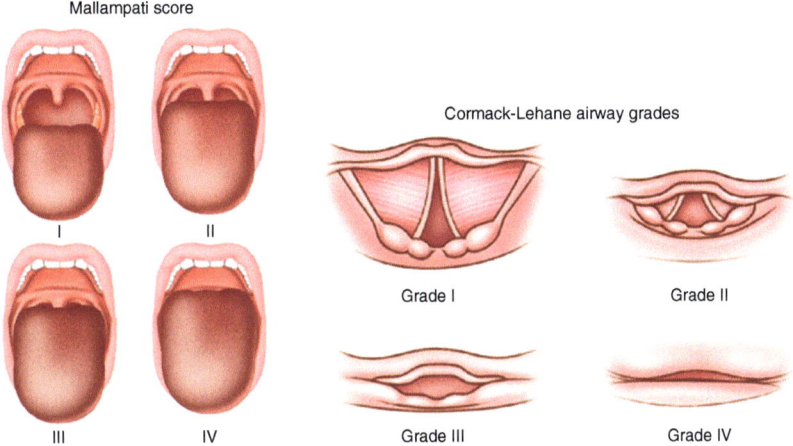

Mallampati score

I   II

III   IV

Cormack-Lehane airway grades

Grade I   Grade II

Grade III   Grade IV

Adapted from: Mallampati SR, Gatt SP, Gugino LD, et al. A clinical sign to predict dif fi cult tracheal intubation: a prospective study. Can Anaesth Soc J 1985;32:429–34

Adapted from: Cormack RS, Lehane J. Dif fi cult tracheal intubation in obstetrics. Cormack-Lehane Airway Grades Anaesthesia 1984; 39: 1105–11

Ventilation Equipment

Bag valve mask devices (anesthesia bag vs. self-inflating bag)
   Suctioning
   Laryngoscope

1. Miller: Straight (<1 year of age)
2. MacIntosh: curved

   Endotracheal tubes

- (Age in years/4) + 4 = ETT size
- Cuffed tubes may be used on all ages.

Chapter 2
Respiratory Review: A, B, C, and P of Kids (Asthma, Bronchiolitis, Croup, and Pneumonia)

Cristina M. Zeretzke-Bien

Abstract Asthma, bronchiolitis, and croup are the ABC diagnoses of the pediatric patient presenting with a respiratory complaint. This chapter highlights the evidence-based care for these specific entities, with associated helpful clinical decision scores to guide care and resource utilization. It also includes the clinical manifestations of pneumonia with age-based antibiotic therapy.

Respiratory Overview

- Children have unique airway anatomy.
- Airway assessment begins with a good history.

  First impressions give *a lot* of information.

Signs of Respiratory Distress

1. Increased work of breathing
2. Altered mental status
3. Color
4. Position
5. Auscultation findings

C. M. Zeretzke-Bien (✉)
Division of Pediatric Emergency Medicine, University of Florida, Gainesville, FL, USA
e-mail: zeretzke@ufl.edu

© The Author(s), under exclusive license to Springer Nature Switzerland AG 2023
C. M. Zeretzke-Bien, T. B. Swan (eds.), *Quick Hits for Pediatric Emergency Medicine*, https://doi.org/10.1007/978-3-031-32650-9_2

Asthma

Asthma is a lower airway disease, which may be chronic or recurrent, with:

- Bronchospasm
- Airway inflammation
- Ventilation problem with air trapping

Clinical Presentation

- Dyspnea
- Retractions
- Tachypnea
- Nasal flaring
- Inability to speak
- Wheezing
- Prolonged expiratory phase
- Beware of the quiet chest

Treatment

- ABCs
- Give oxygen
- Nebulized or MDI beta-agonists (albuterol)
- Ipratropium bromide (Atrovent)
- Steroids
- Upright position
- Severe exacerbation

  - Continuous nebulized therapy
  - Epinephrine (IM or IV)
  - Magnesium sulfate (50 mg/kg, max dose = 2 g)

Considerations for Severe Asthma

- Bolus of fluid
- Baseline BMP to determine K+ as multiple neb treatments can drive K+ into the cell.
- X-ray if other etiology is of concerns (not all that wheezes is asthma).
- Noninvasive positive pressure
- Heliox

Asthma Pearls

- Many patients/parents do not take this disease seriously.
- Parents may not have an asthma action plan.
- Albuterol is a short-acting agent.
- If a patient is requiring multiple albuterol treatments at home, they need immediate evaluation.

Pediatric Asthma Score

Characteristic	0	1	2
Respiratory rate			
2–3 years	<34	35–59	>40
4–5 years	<30	31–35	>36
6–12 years	<26	27–30	>31
>12 years	<23	24–27	>28
Oxygen requirement	<93%	89–92%	<89%
Auscultation	Clear breath sounds	Expiratory wheezes	Inspiratory and expiratory wheezes
Work of breathing	<1 accessory muscle	2 accessory muscles	>3 accessory muscles
Dyspnea	Speaks full sentences, playful, and takes PO well	Speaks partial sentences, short cry, or poor PO	Speaks short phrases, grunting, or unable to PO

Score: 0–3 mild exacerbation, 4–7 moderate exacerbation, 8–10 severe exacerbation

Bronchiolitis

- Lower airway disease
- Airway urgency
- 2 months–2 years
- Chronically ill children are at higher risk:

  - Premature
  - Children with congenital heart disease
  - Less than 1 month of age

- Inflammation, edema, and mucous in the lower airways
- Viral etiology

Clinical Presentation

- Dyspnea
- Tachypnea
- Retractions
- Nasal flaring
- Wheezing
- Long expiratory phase
- Rales
- Rhonchi
- Decreased air movement

Treatment

Supportive

- Oxygen
- Suctioning
- Upright positioning
- High-flow oxygen therapy
- If clinical bronchiolitis, recommendations do not support using albuterol, steroids, chest X-rays, or obtaining other labs.

Bronchiolitis Score

Score	Breath rate	Retractions	Nasal flaring	Wheezing	General status
0	<30	No	No	No	Normal
1	30–45	Only intercostal	Mild and rarely	Heard only with stethoscope	Moderately uneasy and occasionally crying
2	45–60	Intercostal, subcostal, and supraclavicular	Moderately severe and intermittently	Heard in both expiration and inspiration with stethoscope	Very uneasy, crying continuously
3	>60	Abdominal Respiration accompanying Crying	Severe and continuously	Heard in both expiration and inspiration without stethoscope	Lethargic

Croup (Laryngotracheobronchitis)

- Upper laryngotracheobronchitis airway disease
- You will hear *stridor*: *inspiratory*.
- Viral infection of the larynx, trachea, and bronchi

  - Parainfluenza
  - Influenza
  - RSV
  - Adenovirus

- Age 6 months–3 years.
- Male > female
- Winter months

Clinical Presentation

- Fever
- Rhinorrhea
- Barking cough
- Inspiratory stridor
- Respiratory distress
- Worse at night

Clinical Presentation with the Following

- Gradual onset of URI symptoms
- Mild fever, hoarseness, barking cough
- Sudden stridor and retractions
- Dyspnea and tachypnea

Treatment

- Labs and X-rays are unnecessary.
- Mist therapy
- Racemic epinephrine
- Dexamethasone 0.6 mg/kg (maximum dose 16 mg)

Westley Score

	0	1	2	3
Stridor	None	Only with agitation	Mild at rest	Severe at rest
Retraction	None	Mild	Moderate	Severe
Air entry	Normal	Moderate Decrease	Moderate decrease	Marked decrease
Color	Normal	N/A	N/A	Cyanotic
Level of consciousness	Normal	Restless when disturbed	Restless when undisturbed	Lethargic

Score: ≤2 mild croup, 3–5 moderate croup, 6–11 severe croup (consider impending respiratory failure ≥12)

Pneumonia

- Lower airway disease
- Airway urgency
- All ages
- Younger patients can be very ill.
- Chronically ill at higher risk
- Bacterial or viral etiology

Clinical Presentation

- Rales (may be localized).
- Rhonchi
- Tachypnea
- Variable fever
- +/− respiratory distress
- Hypoxemia

Treatment

- Oxygen
- Fluids
- Upright position
- Antibiotic therapy

Pediatric Pneumonia

Age	Bugs	Drugs
Age <5 years	*S. pneumoniae, H. influenzae, Mycoplasma,* group A streptococcus, *C. pneumoniae, S. aureus,* viral, influenza	*PO*: High-dose amoxicillin ± azithromycin (atypical coverage) Alt: Clindamycin, amoxicillin/clavulanate, cefdinir *IV*: Ampicillin ± azithromycin Alt: Ceftriaxone ± azithromycin Add vancomycin or clindamycin if severe illness or features suggestive of *S. aureus* (cavitation, pleural effusion) *Treatment, 10 days Atypical organisms (*Mycoplasma, Chlamydia*) are more common in children >5 years old
Age >5 years and immunized	*S. pneumoniae, Mycoplasma,* group A streptococcus, *C. pneumoniae, S. aureus,* viral, influenza	*PO*: High-dose amoxicillin + azithromycin (atypical coverage) Alt: Clindamycin + azithromycin *IV*: Ampicillin + azithromycin Alt: Ceftriaxone or cefotaxime + azithromycin Add vancomycin or clindamycin if severe illness or features suggestive of *S. aureus* (cavitation, pleural effusion) *Treatment, 7–10 days
Age >5 years and unimmunized for *H. influenzae or S. pneumoniae*	*S. pneumoniae, Mycoplasma,* group A streptococcus, *C. pneumoniae, S. aureus,* viral, influenza	Ceftriaxone or cefotaxime ± azithromycin Add vancomycin or clindamycin if severe illness or features suggestive of *S. aureus* (cavitation, pleural effusion)

Pearls of Pediatric Respiratory Illnesses: Clinical/X-ray/Treatment

Pediatric respiratory illness	Clinical findings	X-ray findings	Treatments
Croup	Barky cough or stridor	Steeple sign	Oral steroids: dexamethasone 0.6 mg/kg Racemic epinephrine if stridor at rest
Asthma	Wheezing	Hyperinflated lungs, flattened diaphragms	1. Oral or IV steroids: dexamethasone or prednisolone 2. Albuterol/atrovent-bronchodilators MDI (spacer) or nebulization 3. Magnesium sulfate IV 4. Continuous albuterol neb
Bronchiolitis	Crackles or expiratory wheeze	RSV—bronchiolitis Presents with RUL atelectasis	Suction High-flow oxygen Consider hypertonic saline nebulized treatment
Pneumonia "Walking pneumonia" or Mycoplasma pneumonia	Crackles bilaterally	Perihilar infiltrate	Antibiotics: azithromycin Oxygen if hypoxic

Pneumonia Focal or community acquired pneumonia	Focal rhonchi	Focal area of consolidation	Antibiotics
			  Oral: high-dose Amoxil 80–90 mg/kg PO BID X 10 days
			Inpatient
			  Ampicillin 50 mg/kg IV q 8
			  Oxygen if hypoxic

Chapter 3
Pediatric Resuscitation

Nishil Patel, Sakina H. Sojar, and Cristina M. Zeretzke-Bien

Abstract This chapter provides easy to follow algorithms to manage the most acutely ill children presenting to the emergency department, including those presenting in cardiac arrest (Lavonas et al., Highlights of the 2020 American Heart Association guidelines for CPR and ECC. Heart.org, Dallas, 2020; Fleegler et al., UpToDate. Wolters Kluwer Health, Philadelphia, 2022). Helpful tips such as reminders of how to perform high quality CPR and medication dosing for common resuscitation medications are embedded into these flow charts. Also featured is emphasis on administration of epinephrine within 5 min in asystole/PEA arrests and ensuring administration of breaths every 2–3 s with a definitive airway as noted in the 2020 American Heart Association Updates, as well as considerations for termination of resuscitation (Lavonas et al., Highlights of the 2020 American Heart Association guidelines for CPR and ECC. Heart.org, Dallas, 2020; American College of Surgeons Committee on Trauma, Ann Emerg Med 63(4):504–515, 2014).

N. Patel
Department of Emergency Medicine, University of Florida Health, Gainesville, FL, USA
e-mail: nishil1patel09@ufl.edu

S. H. Sojar (✉)
Division of Pediatric Emergency Medicine, Department of Emergency Medicine, Warren Alpert Medical School of Brown University, Providence, RI, USA
e-mail: sakina.sojar@brownphysicians.org

C. M. Zeretzke-Bien
Division of Pediatric Emergency Medicine, University of Florida, Gainesville, FL, USA
e-mail: zeretzke@ufl.edu

Pediatric Cardiac Arrest

Start High Quality CPR
- Attach defibrillator pads
- Oxygenate, stalling with 100% FIO2
- No advanced airway? 15:2 compressions to ventilations
- With advanced airway, continuous compressions, breath every 2-3 sec
- Rate 100-120, push ≥1/3 AP diameter of chest, allow for recoil

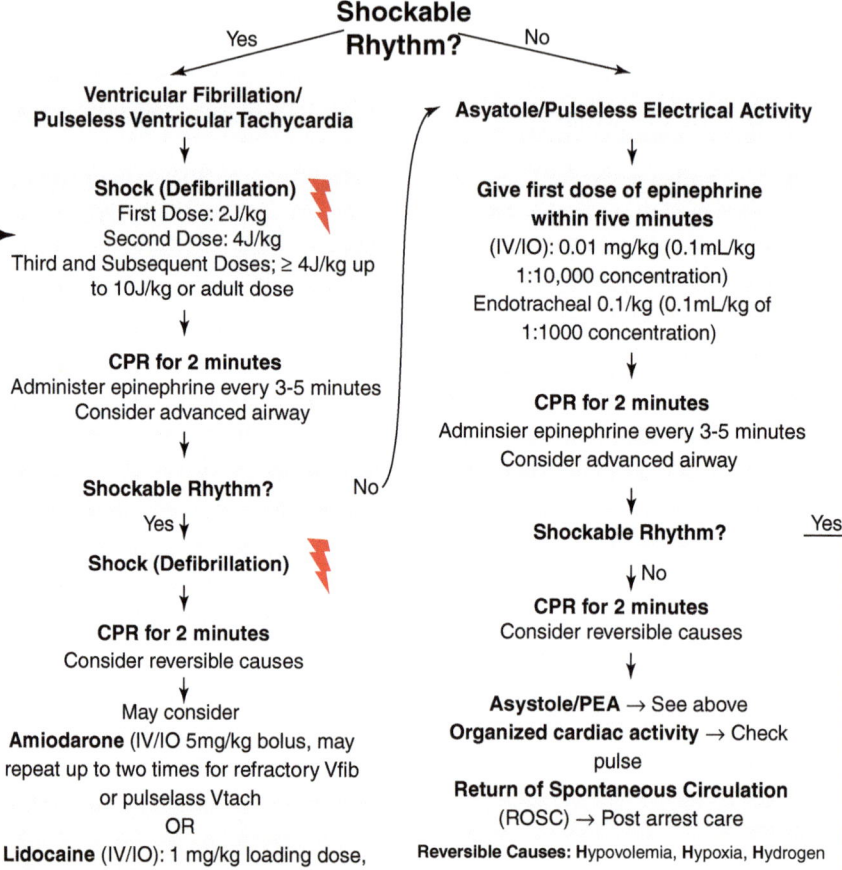

Shockable Rhythm?

Yes → **Ventricular Fibrillation/ Pulseless Ventricular Tachycardia**

No → **Asyatole/Pulseless Electrical Activity**

Shock (Defibrillation)
First Dose: 2J/kg
Second Dose: 4J/kg
Third and Subsequent Doses; ≥ 4J/kg up to 10J/kg or adult dose

CPR for 2 minutes
Administer epinephrine every 3-5 minutes
Consider advanced airway

Shockable Rhythm?   No
Yes

Shock (Defibrillation)

CPR for 2 minutes
Consider reversible causes

May consider
Amiodarone (IV/IO 5mg/kg bolus, may repeat up to two times for refractory Vfib or pulselass Vtach
OR
Lidocaine (IV/IO): 1 mg/kg loading dose, followed dy 20-50 mcg/kg/min Infusion, may repeat bolus after 15 min If needed

Give first dose of epinephrine within five minutes
(IV/IO): 0.01 mg/kg (0.1mL/kg 1:10,000 concentration)
Endotracheal 0.1/kg (0.1mL/kg of 1:1000 concentration)

CPR for 2 minutes
Adminsier epinephrine every 3-5 minutes
Consider advanced airway

Shockable Rhythm?   Yes
No

CPR for 2 minutes
Consider reversible causes

Asystole/PEA → See above
Organized cardiac activity → Check pulse
Return of Spontaneous Circulation (ROSC) → Post arrest care

Reversible Causes: Hypovolemia, Hypoxia, Hydrogen Ion (acidosis), Hypoglycemia, Hypo/Hyperkalemia, Hypothermia, Tension Pneumothorax, Tamponade, Toxins, Thrombosis (pulmonary or coronary)

Pediatric Tachycardia with a Pulse

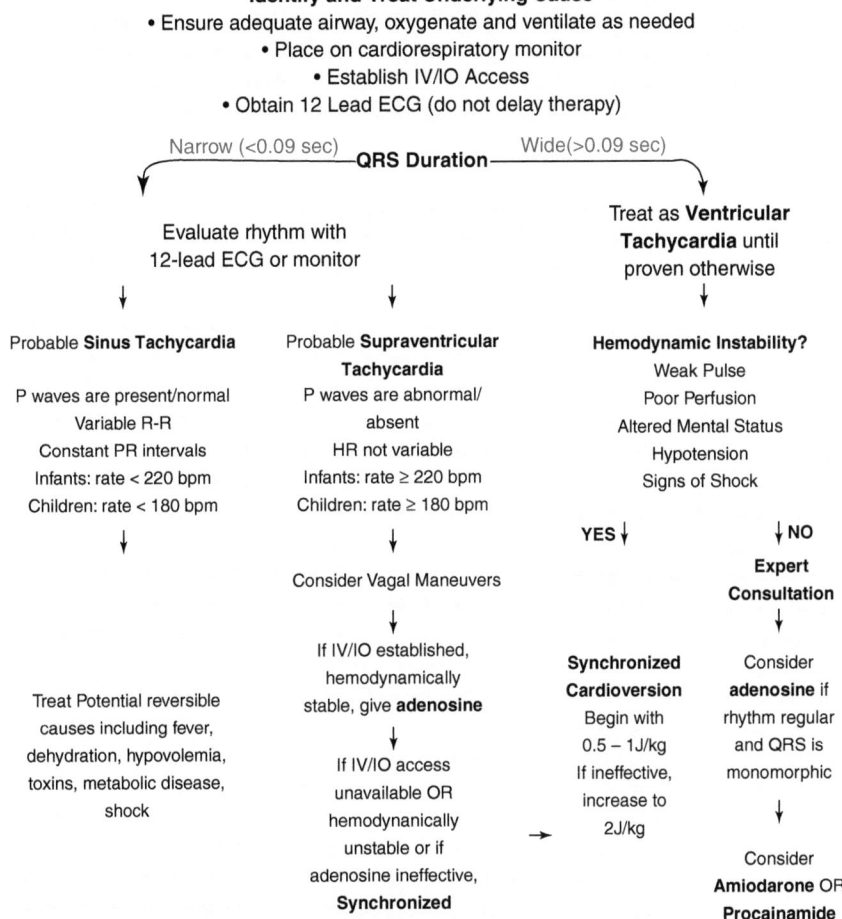

Identify and Treat Underlying Cause
- Ensure adequate airway, oxygenate and ventilate as needed
- Place on cardiorespiratory monitor
- Establish IV/IO Access
- Obtain 12 Lead ECG (do not delay therapy)

Narrow (<0.09 sec) ——**QRS Duration**—— Wide(>0.09 sec)

Evaluate rhythm with
12-lead ECG or monitor

Treat as **Ventricular
Tachycardia** until
proven otherwise

Probable **Sinus Tachycardia**

P waves are present/normal
Variable R-R
Constant PR intervals
Infants: rate < 220 bpm
Children: rate < 180 bpm

Probable **Supraventricular
Tachycardia**
P waves are abnormal/
absent
HR not variable
Infants: rate ≥ 220 bpm
Children: rate ≥ 180 bpm

Hemodynamic Instability?
Weak Pulse
Poor Perfusion
Altered Mental Status
Hypotension
Signs of Shock

YES ↓   **↓ NO**

**Expert
Consultation**

Consider Vagal Maneuvers

Treat Potential reversible
causes including fever,
dehydration, hypovolemia,
toxins, metabolic disease,
shock

If IV/IO established,
hemodynamically
stable, give **adenosine**

If IV/IO access
unavailable OR
hemodynanically
unstable or if
adenosine ineffective,
**Synchronized
Cardioversion**

**Synchronized
Cardioversion**
Begin with
0.5 – 1J/kg
If ineffective,
increase to
2J/kg

Consider
adenosine if
rhythm regular
and QRS is
monomorphic

Consider
Amiodarone OR
Procainamide

Sedation (IV/IM/IO) **(do not delay for comfort):** Lorazepam: 0.1 mg/kg/dose; Midazolam: 0.2 mg/kg/dose
Adenosine (IV/IO) **(rapid bolus):** 1st Dose: 0.1 mg/kg (max 6 mg); 2nd dose: 0.2 mg/kg (max 12 mg)
Amiodarone (IV/IO): 5 mg/kg, administer over 20 - 60 min
Procainamide (IV/IO): 15 mg/kg, administer over 30 - 60 min
(DO NOT routinely administer Amiodarone and Procainamide together)

Pediatric Bradycardia With Poor Perfusion

Identify and Treat Undertying Cause
• Ensure adequate airway, oxygenate and ventilate as needed
• Place on cardiorespiratory monitor
• Establish IV/IO Access
• Obtain 12 Lead ECG (do not delay therapy)

↓

Hemodynamic Instability?
Weak Pulse
Poor Perfusion
Altered Mental Status
Hypotension
Signs of Shock

NO ↓   ↓ **YES**

Support airway, breathing   **Initiate High Quality CPR if Heart**
and circulation   **Rate <60 bpm** with hemodynamic
                                   instability despite adequate
↓   oxygenation and ventilation

Given supplemental oxygen   — **NO**   ↓
                                   Persistent Bradycardia?

                                   ↓ **YES**

Consider expert   **Epinephrine**
consultaiton   (IV/IO): 0.01 mg/kg (0.1mL/kg of
                                   1:10,000 concentration)
                                   Endotracheal 0.1mg/kg (0.1mL/kg of
                                   1:1000 concentration)

                                   ↓

                                   Atropine
                                   (if increased vagal tone or primary
                                   AV block suspected)
                                   (IV/IO) 0.02mg/kg, minimum dose
If pulseless, go to   0.1mg and max dose 0.5mg. May
Pediatric Cardiac   repeat once.
Arrest Algorithm
                                   ↓

                                   Consider transthoracic or
                                   transvenous pacing

Pediatric Septic Shock

Recognition | Presenting Signs Include
Tachycardia (and rarely bradycardia)
Hypotension
Poor perfusion, delayed capillary refill, flash capillary refill
Hyperthermia or hypothermia
Altered mental status
↓

Initial Management
Prioritize airway, breathing and circulation
Place on cardiorespiratory monitor
Establish IV/IO access
Administer 10-20cc/kg isotonic fluid bolus, can repeat with frequent reassessment
Obtain blood cultures and administer broad spectrum antibiotics
Labs: VBG/ABG, poc glucose CBC, BMP, LFT, lactate, ionized calcium
↓

Within the first hour
15-20 minutes ideal

Fluid Refractory Shock?

↓   ↓

Initiation of Vasopressor
Titrate to correct hypotension or poor perfusion
Consider central venous and arterial access

Adrenal insufficiency Risk?
Stress dose Hydrocortisone (IV)
2mg/kg bolus (max 100mg)

↓   ↓

Epinephrine (IV/IO)   **Norepinephrine (IV/IO)**
0.1 to 1 mcg/kg/min   0.1 to 1 mcg/kg/min

Obtain expert consultation with pediatric intensivist

Though reasonable to consider **epinephrine for cold shock** (cold extremities, delayed capillary refill, and/or hypotension) and **norepinephrine for warm shock** (warm extremities, "flash" capillary refill, and/or hypotension) -- time is of the essence, initiate the vasopressor that is most readily available.

Suspected Opioid Overdose

Recognition:
Bradypnea, agonal breathing, or respiratory arrest
Pinpoint pupils
Altered mental status
Decreased consciousness
↓

**Initiate rescue breathing with
bag valve mask ventilation**
↓

Administer Naloxone
(IV/IO/IM/subcutaneous)
0.1 mg/kg, q2min, max dose of 2mg/dose up to a
max of 10mg
↓

Patient breathing normally?

YES ↓   ↓ NO

Provide supportive
care. Place patient on
end-tidal device. Be
prepared to provide
additional doses of
naloxone or initiate a
continuous infusion.

Continue to support
breathing with bag-
valve-mask ventilation.
Administer additional
dose of naloxone.

If patient is pulseless,
initiate high quality
CPR.

Termination of Resuscitation

- No single data point, in isolation, is dependable enough to reliably guide the end of resuscitation [1, 2].
- The decision to terminate resuscitative efforts should be made in the context of each unique patient, their surrounding circumstances, and after considering the following factors: [1]

  - Do not resuscitate status (DNR)
  - Duration of cardiac arrest
  - When was the patient discovered?

  - Time from discovery to CPR initiated?
  - Initial rhythm (i.e. shockable vs. asystole or PEA)
  - Disease state (chronic or terminal conditions, sepsis, respiratory failure, cardiac disease, metabolism errors)

- Likelihood of intact survival after prolonged resuscitation (defined as >30 min) is higher in the following conditions: [1]

  - Hypothermic arrest (e.g. cold water drowning)
  - Poisonings
  - Patients with cardiac disease who were resuscitated with ECPR (ECMO with CPR)
  - Lightning strike or high voltage injury

- In an otherwise futile appearing resuscitation, a provider may consider terminal cessation of resuscitation after a parent/guardian arrives at bedside as this has shown improved emotional and coping outcomes for the caregiver, provided this does not result in unreasonable prolongation of death or unnecessary use of critical resources [1, 2].

References

1. Fleegler E, Kleinman M, Torrey SB. Pediatric advanced life support (PALS). In: UpToDate. Philadelphia: Wolters Kluwer Health; 2022.
2. American College of Surgeons Committee on Trauma. Withholding or termination of resuscitation in pediatric out-of-hospital traumatic cardiopulmonary arrest. Ann Emerg Med. 2014;63(4):504–15. https://doi.org/10.1016/j.annemergmed.2014.01.013.

Chapter 4
Pediatric Pearls: Management of Shock in Children

Nhi Luu and Cristina M. Zeretzke-Bien

Abstract The chapters on resuscitation and shock are incredibly valuable in the undifferentiated shock patient. It will set you up for success with initial stabilization while performing evidence-based care. The assistance with dosing for the common "code drugs" is a valuable reference in a high-anxiety situations like the crashing pediatric patient.

Shock

Defined as abnormal physiologic state in which there is an inability to deliver adequate oxygen to meet the metabolic needs of the body.

Types of shock
Hypovolemic
Cardiogenic
Distributive
Obstructive

- Vitals are extremely variable in pediatric shock. Evaluate the patient.
- Tachycardia is an early finding, while bradycardia is a late finding.
- Tachypnea is an early finding. Widened pulse pressure may be an early subtle finding.
- Prompt recognition of shock is important for aggressive treatment.

N. Luu
Department of Emergency Medicine, University of Florida, Gainesville, FL, USA
e-mail: nluu@ufl.edu

C. M. Zeretzke-Bien (✉)
Division of Pediatric Emergency Medicine, University of Florida, Gainesville, FL, USA
e-mail: zeretzke@ufl.edu

© The Author(s), under exclusive license to Springer Nature Switzerland AG 2023
C. M. Zeretzke-Bien, T. B. Swan (eds.), *Quick Hits for Pediatric Emergency Medicine*, https://doi.org/10.1007/978-3-031-32650-9_4

- More than one type of shock may be present.

$$\text{Cardiac Output}\,(\text{CO}) = \text{Heart Rate}\,(\text{HR}) \times \text{Stoke Volume}\,(\text{SV})$$

Quick Hit Cardiac Pearls

Cardiac output (CO) is the amount of blood the heart pumps through the circulatory system in a minute. Children compensate for cardiac output with increased heart rates. Children tolerate high heart rates.

Hypovolemic Shock

- Most common cause of shock around the world. Most of the time from sensible GI losses.
- Requires aggressive fluid management!
- Treatment is isotonic fluid bolus (20 ml/kg) up to 60–80 ml/kg with two large-bore IVs.
- Consider resuscitation with blood products at 10 mL/kg if signs of bleeding are present and with no improvement with IV fluid boluses.

Cardiogenic Shock:

- Assess for cardiac arrythmias prior to fluid administration
- Use 10 ml/kg isotonic crystalloid fluid bolus.

Septic Shock: The Golden Hour

- Maintain perfusion, oxygenation, and ventilation.
- Inadequate early fluid resuscitation is associated with increased mortality.
- Start empiric antibiotic therapy within 1 h of presentation

Definition of Hypotension by Systolic Blood Pressure and Age

Age	Systolic BP (mmHg)
Term neonates (0–28 days)	<60
Infants (1–12 m)	<70
Children 1–10 years (fifth percentile)	<70 + (age in years × 2)
Children >10	<90

Heart Rate and Perfusion Pressure for Age

Current age	Heart rate	MAP-CVP
Term neonate	120–180	55
<1	120–180	60
<2	120–160	65
<7	100–140	65
<15	90–140	65

Adapted from Carcillo JA, Fields AI, American College of Critical Care Medicine Task Force Committee Members: Clinical practice parameters for hemodynamic support of pediatric and neonatal patients in septic shock. *Crit Care Med.* 2002;30:1371

Pediatric CPR

The most common causes of cardiac arrest in children are respiratory failure and hypotensive shock.

- Emphasis on effective CPR—Most important: *compressions*
- CPR sequence: Chest compressions, airway, breathing
- Depress 1/3 of the anterior–posterior diameter of the chest. Allow full recoil!

  – Approximately 1 1/2 inches in infant
  – Approximately 2 inches in children

- "Push hard, push fast."
- Rate: 100 compressions/minute. Single rescuer: 30:2 (compressions: ventilations).
- Two rescuers trained in CPR: 15:2 (compressions: ventilations). NEW 2020 PALS guideline change! Once intubated, provide continuous compressions with breaths every 2–3 s. Shock energy for defibrillation: First shock 2 J/kg, second shock 4 J/kg, any subsequent shocks >4 J/kg, with maximum 10 J/kg or adult dose.

Pediatric Pearls

Do Not Hyperventilate!

Excessive ventilation increases intrathoracic pressure:

- Decreased cardiac output, cerebral flow, and coronary flow
- Air trapping
- Risk of stomach inflation and aspiration

If patient has perfusion and return of spontaneous circulation (ROSC), but still not breathing or intubated, then ventilation should be 12–20 breaths per minute.

SIRS Criteria

In children, the SIRS criteria are modified and must include at least two of the following:

1. **Heart rate** >2 standard deviations above normal for age in the absence of stimuli such as pain and drug administration or unexplained persistent elevation for greater than 30 min. In infants, it also includes heart rate <10th percentile for age in the absence of vagal stimuli, beta-blockers, or congenital heart disease or unexplained persistent depression for greater than 30 min.
2. **Body temperature** obtained orally, rectally, from Foley temp catheter probe, or from central venous catheter probe <36 °C or >38.5 °C. *Temperature must be abnormal to qualify as SIRS in pediatric patients.*
3. **Respiratory rate** >2 standard deviations above normal for age or the requirement for mechanical ventilation not related to neuromuscular disease *or* the administration of anesthesia.
4. **White blood cell** count elevated or depressed for age not related to chemotherapy or greater than 10% bands.

Common Pediatric Medications for Resuscitation and Cardiac Arrest

Epinephrine

- 0.01 mg/kg of 1:10,000 IV/IO or 0.1 mg/kg of 1:1000 endotracheal (ET). (IV or IO route is preferred.)
- Repeat every 3–5 min as needed.

Atropine

- 0.02 mg/kg IV/IO or 0.04–0.06 mg/kg ET
- *New 2020 update!* Minimum dose 0.1 mg.
- Maximum single dose 0.5 mg
- May repeat once if needed.
- Not used routinely for pre-treatment or sedation

Adenosine

- 0.1 mg/kg IV/IO, followed by 0.2 mg/kg
- Maximum dose 6 mg first dose, 12 mg second dose

Amiodarone

- 5 mg/kg IV/IO bolus, may repeat up to 3 total doses of 15 mg/kg total.
- Maximum dose 300 mg

Lidocaine

- 1 mg/kg loading dose

Procainamide

- 15 mg/kg IV/IO over 30–60 min

Magnesium Sulfate (for Torsades)

- 25–50 mg/kg IV/IO over several minutes
- Maximum dose of 2 g

Chapter 5
Pediatric Ventilator Management

Tricia B. Swan and Carmen J. Martinez

Abstract This is the go-to guide for invasive and noninvasive ventilation for the non-intensivist. From the crashing asthmatic to the patient requiring titration of their ventilator, this chapter sets you up for success in the pre- and post-intubation period for the pediatric respiratory failure patient. The DOPES mnemonic is a quick hit that everyone must know when your ventilated patient acutely deteriorates in order to troubleshoot and quickly correct their decompensation.

T. B. Swan (✉)
Division of Pediatric Emergency Medicine, University of Florida, Gainesville, FL, USA
e-mail: tfalgiani@ufl.edu

C. J. Martinez
Division of Pediatric Emergency Medicine, Department of Emergency Medicine, USA Health Children's and Women's Hospital, University of South Alabama, Mobile, AL, USA
e-mail: cmartinez@health.southalabama.edu

C. M. Zeretzke-Bien, T. B. Swan (eds.), *Quick Hits for Pediatric Emergency Medicine*, https://doi.org/10.1007/978-3-031-32650-9_5

27

Noninvasive Modes of Ventilation

Benefits	Indications	Contraindications
• Reduce work of breathing (Reduce oxygen consumption) • Reverse hypoventilation (Increase tidal volume) • Increase FRC- improve oxygenation, lung compliance • Maintain and splint collapsed airways • Preserved defense mechanisms • Improve diaphragmatic activity • Less sedation	• Respiratory insufficiency • Aspiration • Chronic lung disease • Pulmonary edema • Bronchioilitis • Pneumonia • Status asthmaticus • Obstructive sleep apnea • Neuromuscular diseases (weakness) • Post-extubation respiratory insufficiency	• Severely impaired consciousness • Inability to protect airway • Inability to clear secretions • Craniofacial deformities or injuries • Pneumothorax • Shock • Cardiopulmonary arrest

High-Flow Nasal Cannula	CPAP	BiPAP

• Heated, humidified, high flow oxygen
• Up to 60L/min and 100% FiO_2
• Creates 2-3 cm H_2O of PEEP
• Increases alveolar O_2
• Decreased CO_2
• Reduces deadspace
• Initial setting
  • 1-2 L/kg/min
	• Delivers a fixed positive pressure throughout the respiratory cycle
	• Pressure does not change with inspiration or expiration
	• Initial setting at 5 cm H_2O
	• May increase to 5-8 cm H_2O if poor lung compliance (stiff lungs)
		• Delivers different levels of pressure during inspiration (IPAP) and expiration (EPAP)
		• Increase the EPAP to improve work of breathing and oxygenation
		• Increase the Δ (IPAP-EPAP) to improve ventilation
		• Initial settings:
		  • Infants: 10/5
		  • Children: 12/8

CPAP—continuous positive airway pressure; BiPAP—Bilevel positive airway pressure

Invasive Ventilation

Indications for invasive ventilation:

- Respiratory failure or insufficiency
  - Hypoxia ($PaO_2 < 50$)
  - Hypercarbia ($PaCO_2 > 50$)
- Inability to protect airway (low GCS, excessive secretions, obstruction, inhalation injury)
- Severe respiratory distress
- Increased ICP
- Apnea
- Excessive respiratory load (shock, uncompensated acidosis)

Types of Ventilator Support

Pressure Control	Volume Control
• Gas flow is delivered until a preset pressure is reached and then held for the set I-time • Delivery of reliable set tidal volume difficult: volume of gas delivered is small in relation to volume in the ventilator circuit • Reduces risk of barotrauma • Useful for newborn and infant ventilatory support • Consider pressure control setting for large air leaks due to small ET tube size, poor lung compliance or poor ventilation due to adult size vent circuit on a small infant/child • As lung compliance increases, tidal volume increases • Set pressure control to give effective chest rise and adequate air entry (expect PIPs 18-22 in healthy lungs, 23-27 in moderate lung disease, 28-35 in severe lung disease)	• Preset tidal volume is delivered to patient, regardless of the pressure required • Increased risk for barotrauma • As lung compliance worsens, PIP will increase • Risk of barotrauma can be reduced by pressure alarms and pressure pop-off valves • Adult size ventilator circuits may require you to increase the tidal volume (circuit takes large volume amount itself)

Modes of Ventilation

Mode	Definition	Advantages	Disadvantages
Volume control (assist control or AC/VC)	Each breath is the same flow, volume, and I-time regardless of mandatory or triggered breath	Full ventilator support Controlled minute ventilation Able to measure mechanics	Fixed flow rate and pattern increase risk for asynchrony on the ventilator
Synchronized intermittent mandatory ventilation (SIMV)	Volume or pressure controlled breaths are delivered at a set rate and synchronized with patient trigger. Additional breaths are not controlled	Extra breaths are comfortable Allows the patient to finish expiration before cycling on	Can have rapid shallow breathing if pressure support is not adequate
Pressure support (PSV, CPAP)	Each breath is supported but patient determines the volume, rate, and inspiratory time	Increased patient comfort Patient determines their own minute ventilation	Minute ventilation completely dependent on patient effort Tidal volume can get too low or too high
Pressure control (AC/PC)	Every breath has the same I-time and peak inspiratory pressure regardless of triggered or mandatory breath	Variable flow rate and pattern increase patient comfort Able to limit PIP (important if airway surgery)	If poor patient effort or lung compliance, volume can get too low If increased patient effort or increased lung compliance, volume can get too high

Initial Ventilator Settings

	Infant	Child	Adolescent
Tidal volume	7–10 mL/kg	7–10 mL/kg	7–10 mL/kg
Respiratory rate	25–30 bpm	15–20 bpm	8–12 bpm
PEEP	5 cm H_2O	5 cm H_2O	5 cm H_2O
FiO_2	Start at 100% and wean to avoid oxygen toxicity Goal: sats >90%	Start at 100% and wean to avoid oxygen toxicity Goal: sats >90%	Start at 100% and wean to avoid oxygen toxicity Goal: sats >90%
Inspiratory time (I-time)	0.5 s[a]	0.7–0.8 s[a]	0.8–1.0 s[a]
PIP	<30 cm H_2O, use minimal pressure needed to produce adequate chest wall movement (usually <25 cm H_2O if normal lungs)	<30 cm H_2O, use minimal pressure needed to produce adequate chest wall movement (usually <25 cm H_2O if normal lungs)	<30 cm H_2O, use minimal pressure needed to produce adequate chest wall movement (usually <25 cm H_2O if normal lungs)

[a] In asthma shorten the I-time to allow more time for expiration to overcome air trapping

DOPES

Troubleshooting a ventilated patient that acutely deteriorates (acute hypoxemia or cardiovascular collapse)

D: Displaced ETT—check for equal BS, $EtCO_2$, CXR.

O: Obstructed airway—suction patient, mucous plug, replace ETT.

P: Pneumothorax—check for equal BS, needle decompression, bedside ultrasound for pleural sliding, CXR.

E: Equipment failure—disconnect from circuit, hand ventilate, ensure 100% FIO_2 is flowing.

S: Stacking/stretching (breaths stacking in asthma, over-PEEP in non-recruitable lung segments) —disconnect from circuit, compress chest, allow full exhalation, decrease RR, decrease PEEP, decrease tidal volume.

Quick Hit Pediatric Ventilator Management Pearls

1. Pediatric patients have higher resistance due to narrower airways, as well as high chest-wall compliance. A more pliable chest wall results in lower functional residual capacity.
2. Cuffed endotracheal tubes are now preferred to uncuffed endotracheal tubes in most circumstances.
3. Use synchronized intermittent mandatory ventilation (SIMV) for patients without spontaneous respiratory effort and use SIMV with pressure support for patients with spontaneous respiratory effort.
4. In patients with asthma, please remember to set a low respiratory rate and shorten the inspiration time (I time) to allow for full exhalation and prevent air trapping.

Chapter 6
Neonatal Delivery and the Acutely Ill Neonate

Tricia B. Swan and Juan Carlos Gonzalez

Abstract The sick or crashing neonate is a stressful patient for any emergency provider. THE MISFITS mnemonic is a must-know heuristic for the potential causes of severe illness in patients under 28 days of age. A quick review of the latest phototherapy guidelines for hyperbilirubinemia is included! The steps for the precipitous delivery of the newborn are a quick-glance guide to review prior to that EMS arrival. The newborn resuscitation medication flowcharts and the umbilical vein catheter (UVC) placement procedure checklist are some of the top "Quick Hits" in this book.

Neonates (Age ≤28 days)

Causes of severe illness in neonates: THE MISFITS

T	Trauma/non-accidental trauma (abuse)
H	Heart disease (ductal-dependent congenital lesions)
E	Endocrine and electrolyte disorders
M	Metabolic disorders (congenital adrenal hyperplasia, thyrotoxicosis)
I	Inborn errors of metabolism
S	Sepsis
F	Formula miscalculation (dilution or over concentration)
I	Intestinal catastrophes (volvulus, NEC, intussusception)
T	Toxins (home remedies)
S	Seizures

T. B. Swan
Division of Pediatric Emergency Medicine, University of Florida, Gainesville, FL, USA
e-mail: tfalgiani@ufl.edu

J. C. Gonzalez (✉)
Division of Pediatric Emergency Medicine, Department of Emergency Medicine, UF Health Shands Children's Hospital, University of Florida College of Medicine, Gainesville, FL, USA
e-mail: Juan.gonzalez@ufl.edu

Immediate evaluation and treatment of the critically ill neonate includes

1. ABCs
2. IV fluids (10–20 cc/kg)
3. Bedside glucose

    (a) Treat hypoglycemia 2–4 mL/kg of D10
    (b) Follow with continuous dextrose infusion at 5–8 mg/kg/min

4. Initiation of antibiotic therapy to treat for presumed sepsis/meningitis

    (a) Ampicillin + gentamicin IV OR
    (b) Ampicillin + ceftazidime IV

5. Head CT if seizures or suspect trauma (including abuse)
6. Prostaglandin for ductal-dependent congenital heart lesions

    (a) Apnea is a side effect of prostaglandin—be prepared to intubate.
    (b) Start infusion at 0.05 mcg/kg/min and may gradually increase to 0.4 mcg/kg/min.

7. Steroids for congenital adrenal hyperplasia

    (a) Give hydrocortisone 25 mg IV

8. If seizures:

    (a) Correct hypoglycemia
    (b) Phenobarbital 20 mg/kg IV loading dose
    (c) Pyridoxine 100 mg IV

9. Labs to obtain when possible (**not the primary goal; please give fluids, meds, and critical interventions first; may obtain labs and cultures at a later time): CBC, CMP, blood culture, UA, urine culture, CSF studies and CSF culture, lactate, ammonia, serum amino acids, urine organic acids

Newborn Delivery and Resuscitation (Fig. 6.1)

MR SOPA Ventilation Correction Steps

M	Mask reposition
R	Reposition airway (sniffing position)
S	Suction mouth then nose
O	Open mouth and airway
P	Pressure increase (increase PEEP on BVM)
A	Artificial airway (ETT or LMA)

Endotracheal intubation guide

Baby's weight	Gestational age	ET tube size
<1 kg	<28 weeks	2.5
1–2 kg	29–34 weeks	3.0
2–3 kg	34–38 weeks	3.5
>3 kg	>38 weeks	3.5–4.0

Airway	Breathing	Circulation	Drugs
• Suction mouth then nose • Head placement in sniffing position	• HR <100, apnea or poor effort: give PPV at 40-60 BPM • Observe for rise in HR for 15 seconds of PPV • If no rise in HR or chest not moving: perform MR SOPA corrective steps until chest rise • Attach pulse ox and cardiac monitor • Intubate or LMA placement and give PPV for 30 seconds before starting compressions	• Compressions if HR < 60 BPM after 30 seconds of PPV with good chest movement • Check HR every 1 minute • 3 compressions: 1 breath • Use 100% oxygen • Use cardiac monitor to assess HR during CPR (not brachial or umbilical pulse)	• If HR < 60 BPM after 1 min of CPR: Give epinephrine • May give epinephrine via ETT, IV, IO, UVC • Repeat every 3-5 minutes if HR < 60 BPM with compressions

*PPV = positive pressure ventilation, HR = heart rate

Fig. 6.1 Newborn delivery and resuscitation

UVC Placement

Supplies needed

1. Sterile gowns, gloves, towels, and drapes
2. Antiseptic solution
3. 3.5 French umbilical catheter for infants <1500 g or 5 French umbilical catheter for infants >1500 g (may use 5 French feeding tube in place of umbilical catheter in emergent situation)
4. 10 mL syringe with heparinized saline flush and three-way stopcock
5. Umbilical tape (or suture material)
6. Non-toothed forceps, small hemostats, and #11 scalpel

   Procedure (Figs. 6.2 and 6.3)

1. Prepare and drape for sterile placement. Clean the skin and umbilical cord with antiseptic solution.
2. Loosely tie umbilical tape or suture at the base of the umbilical stump.
3. Using a scalpel, cut the umbilical cord horizontally approximately 3–4 cm from the skin.
4. Identify the two arteries and one vein. The two arteries are thick walled and smaller than the vein. The vein is thin walled with a larger lumen.
5. Place UVC catheter into the umbilical vein and advance the catheter approximately 2 cm beyond the point in which good blood flow is obtained. Emergency UVC access is 5 cm +length of umbilical stump.
6. Loosen umbilical tape if resistance if met; otherwise, tighten tape after UVC is passed.
7. Secure catheter placement and obtain X-ray for placement confirmation.

APGAR Scores

Note: APGAR scores are to denote the physiologic state of the neonate at that singular point in time. It does not predict future mortality or morbidity. APGAR should be noted at 1 min and 5 min

Sign	0 point	1 point	2 points
A—Activity	Absent, flaccid limp	Flexed arms and legs	Active movement
P—Pulse	Absent	Below 100 bpm	Over 100 bpm
G—Grimace	Floppy	Minimal response to stimulation	Strong response to stimulation
A—Appearance	Blue or pale	Pink body, blue extremities	Pink
R—Respirations	Absent	Slow or irregular	Vigorous cry

Severely depressed	0–3
Moderately depressed	4–6
Excellent condition	7–10

Hyperbilirubinemia

Jaundice within the first 24 h of life is pathologic. Jaundice presenting after the first 24 h of life requires investigation to see if the neonate needs phototherapy. For evaluation of jaundice, please obtain both direct and indirect bilirubin levels.

Below are the updated phototherapy thresholds for neonates presenting with jaundice. Once a newborn is above the line for therapy, it is recommended patient be started on phototherapy. The goal of neonatal hyperbilirubinemia management is to prevent neurotoxicity, encephalopathy, and kernicterus.

• Neurotoxic risk factors (Figs. 6.4 and 6.5)

  – Preterm gestation (gestational age <38 weeks)
  – Red blood cell disorders, including G6PD deficiency
  – Albumin <3.0 g/dL
  – Sepsis
  – Isoimmune hemolytic disease (Coombs positive)
  – Clinical instability in the prior 24 h

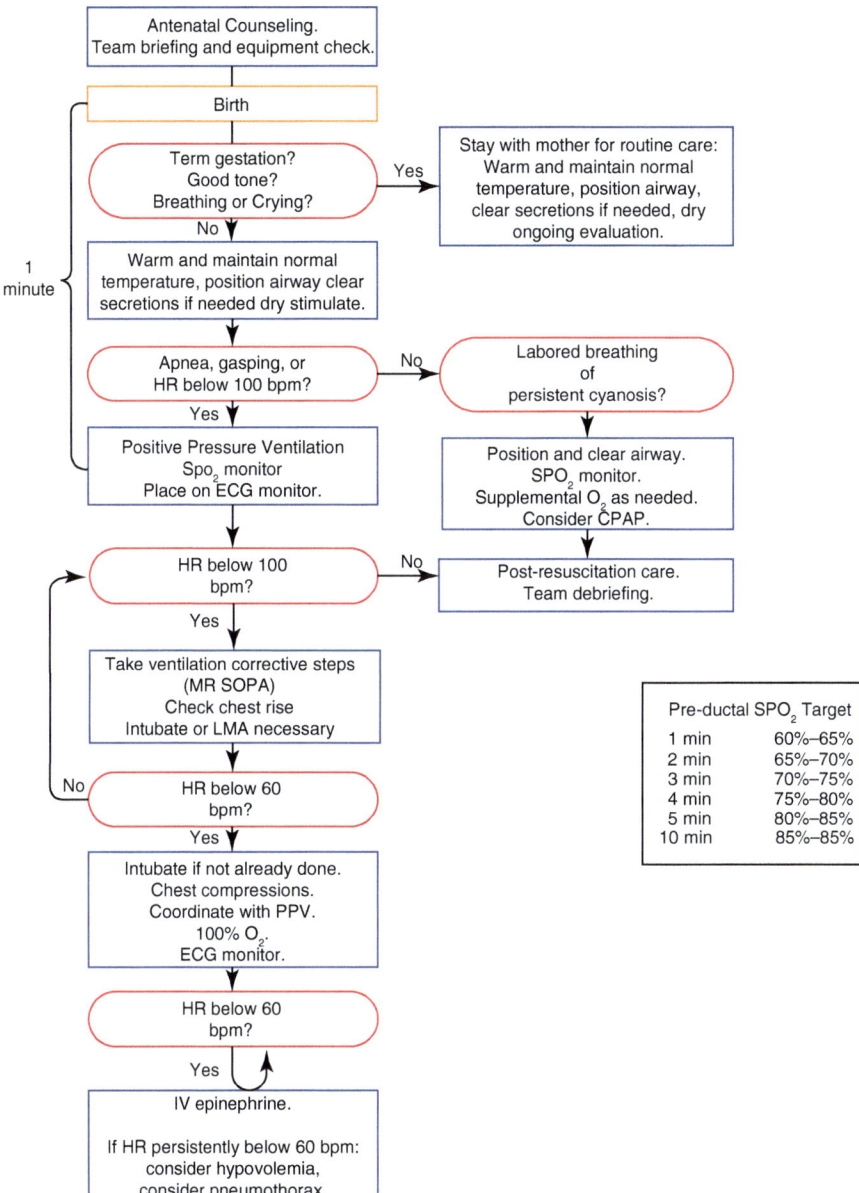

Fig. 6.2 Neonatal resuscitation algorithm

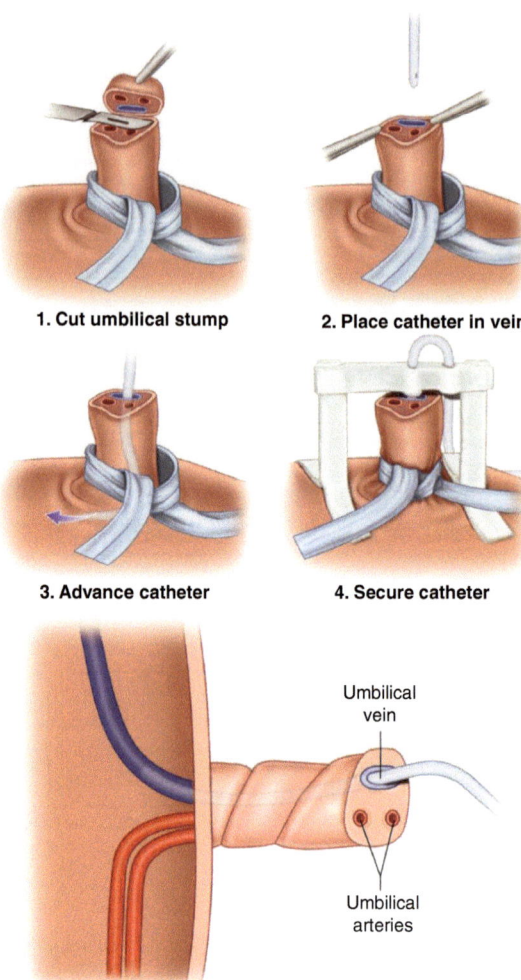

1. Cut umbilical stump

2. Place catheter in vein

3. Advance catheter

4. Secure catheter

Umbilical vein

Umbilical arteries

Fig. 6.3 Umbilical venous catheter (UVC) placement

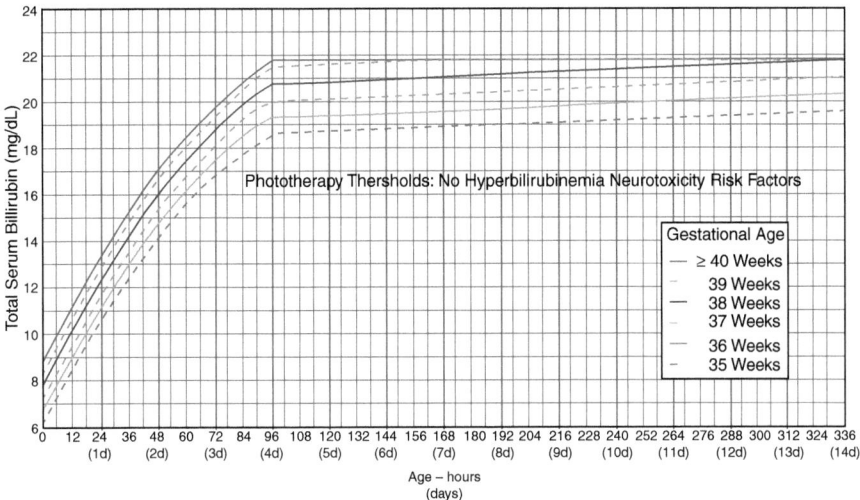

Fig. 6.4 Phototherapy threshold with no risk factors

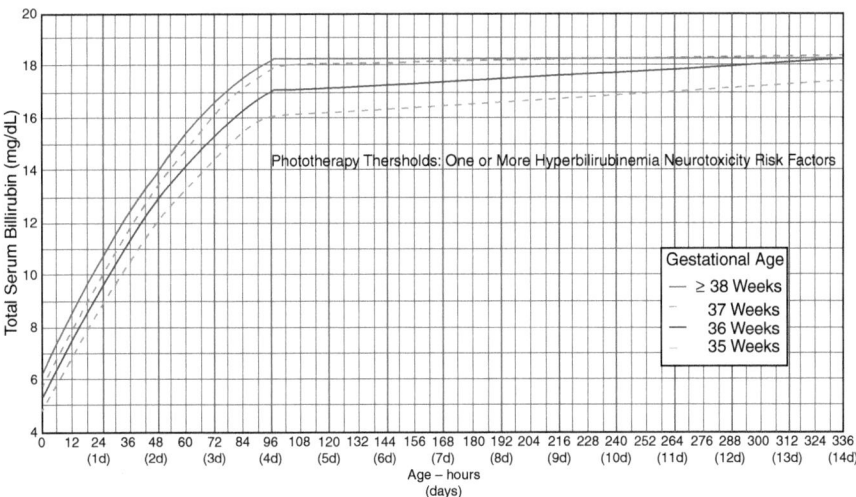

Fig. 6.5 Phototherapy threshold with >1 risk factor

Quick Hits Neonatal Delivery and the Acutely Ill Neonate Pearls

1. The differential for a severely ill neonate is large—use THE MISFITS mnemonic to help you identify causes and start treatment immediately.
2. Apnea is a side effect of treatment with prostaglandin—be ready to intubate!
3. Resuscitation of the newly born infant with signs of distress (apnea, gasping, or heart rate <100 BPM) always begins with proper airway management and adequate breaths delivered by positive pressure ventilation.
4. Evaluation of hyperbilirubinemia in neonates requires both direct and indirect bilirubin levels.

Chapter 7
Pediatric Abdominal Pain

**Sadiqa A. I. Kendi, Victoria M. Wurster Ovalle,
and Cristina M. Zeretzke-Bien**

Abstract Abdominal emergencies differ by age in the pediatric population. This chapter is a wonderful way to frame the likelihood of a diagnosis in an easy-to-read table format packed with "Quick Hits." The pearls at the end of the chapter are a nice way to avoid some common pitfalls in the pediatric patient with abdominal pain.

Common Diagnoses with Work-Up and Management

Symptoms	Diagnosis to consider	Work-Up	Management
Right lower quadrant pain, fever, vomiting	Appendicitis	Ultrasound (CT only if unable to visualize), complete blood count (CBC), C-reactive protein (CRP)	Appendectomy
Bilious vomiting in an infant	Malrotation with volvulus	Abdominal X-ray "double bubble sign," upper GI series	NG placement, IV fluid resuscitation, and operative management (Ladd procedure)

S. A. I. Kendi
Pediatric Emergency Medicine, Children's National Health System, Washington, DC, USA
e-mail: skendi@cnmc.org

V. M. Wurster Ovalle (✉)
Pediatric Emergency Medicine, Nemours Children's Hospital, Orlando, FL, USA
e-mail: victoria.wursterovalle@nemours.org

C. M. Zeretzke-Bien
Division of Pediatric Emergency Medicine, University of Florida, Gainesville, FL, USA
e-mail: zeretzke@ufl.edu

C. M. Zeretzke-Bien, T. B. Swan (eds.), *Quick Hits for Pediatric Emergency Medicine*, https://doi.org/10.1007/978-3-031-32650-9_7

41

Symptoms	Diagnosis to consider	Work-Up	Management
Vomiting and intermittent abdominal pain in infant (bloody stool is a late sign)	Intussusception	Ultrasound (US)	IV fluids, air enema (diagnostic and therapeutic)
Right upper quadrant pain which is colicky	Cholelithiasis	US	Pain management, delayed operative management
Right upper quadrant pain which is colicky with fever	Cholecystitis	US	Antibiotics
Epigastric pain radiating to back, vomiting	Pancreatitis	Labs (lipase, amylase)	Bowel rest, fluids
Painless rectal bleeding	Meckel's diverticulum	Meckel's scan	Operative management (surgical resection)
Lower quadrant abdominal pain with vaginal bleeding	Ectopic pregnancy	Quantitative HCG, pelvic US, type, and screen	Surgical resection or methotrexate (medical therapy)
Vaginal discharge, lower abdominal pain	Pelvic inflammatory disease	Bimanual exam, sed rate (ESR), C-reactive protein (CRP), US if concerned about Fitz-Hugh-Curtis	Antibiotics
Lower quadrant abdominal pain, colicky	Ovarian torsion	Pelvic US	Operative management (detorsion or oophorectomy)
Nonbilious projectile emesis in infant <2 months old	Pyloric stenosis	Abdominal US, electrolytes	IV fluids, correct electrolytes, operative management (pyloromyotomy)
Generalized crampy abdominal pain	Constipation	None; rule out other possible diagnoses	Laxatives, fiber, water
Flank pain, colicky	Renal stones	Renal US to evaluate for hydronephrosis, urinalysis to rule out infected stone, CT without contrast to further evaluate	Fluids, pain control, operative management with urology for obstructive stone

Differential Diagnosis for Abdominal Pain Stratified by Age

Infant	Toddler	Child	Adolescent
Pyloric stenosis	**Malrotation with volvulus**	Appendicitis	Testicular torsion
Malrotation with volvulus	**Appendicitis**	Testicular torsion	Ovarian torsion
Gastroesophageal reflux disease	**Testicular torsion**	Pancreatitis	**Ectopic pregnancy**
Urinary tract infection	Meckel's diverticulum	Acute gastroenteritis	Pelvic inflammatory disease
Non-accidental trauma	**Non-accidental trauma**	**Diabetic ketoacidosis**	Pancreatitis
Acute gastroenteritis	Acute gastroenteritis	Constipation	Cholelithiasis
Necrotizing enterocolitis	Constipation	**Pneumonia**	Cholecystitis
Hirschsprung's disease	Intussusception	Hemolytic uremic syndrome	Peptic ulcer disease
Incarcerated hernia	**Increased intracranial pressure**	Porphyria	Appendicitis
Increased intracranial pressure	**Pneumonia**	Pharyngitis	Acute gastroenteritis
Myocarditis	**Myocarditis**	Myocarditis	**Diabetic ketoacidosis**
Colic	Foreign body/toxic ingestion		Inflammatory bowel disease (IBD)
			Irritable bowel syndrome (IBS)

Easy-to-miss diagnoses in bold

Quick Hits Abdominal Pain Pearls

1. Abdominal pain and vomiting in kids doesn't always equate to an intraabdominal process. Always do a complete physical exam and consider lower lobe pneumonia, testicular torsion, and intracranial processes (atypical diagnoses that can present with vomiting and abdominal pain).
2. Classic electrolyte abnormalities in pyloric stenosis are hypochloremia, hypokalemia, and metabolic alkalosis.
3. Classic "currant jelly stools" are only seen in about 50% of intussusception cases.
4. Ultrasound, when available, is the preferred imaging modality in children to diagnose appendicitis, intussusception, pyloric stenosis, and torsion.

Chapter 8
Trauma Tidbits

Cristina M. Zeretzke-Bien and Joon Choi

Abstract Pediatric trauma is the #1 etiology of morbidity and mortality in the US pediatric population. This chapter is a great assist with appropriate dosing, fluids, and the ABCDEs of resuscitation. The modified Glasgow Coma Scale (GCS) for age is always a challenge to remember but is right there as the first item of the chapter for easy reference.

Glasgow Coma Scale

Trauma score	Motor activity	Verbal activity	Eye opening
1	None	None	None
2	Extension to pain	Incomprehensible	To pain
3	Flexion to pain	Inappropriate	To command
4	Withdraws to pain	Confused	Spontaneous
5	Localizes pain	Oriented	–
6	Obeys commands		–

C. M. Zeretzke-Bien
Division of Pediatric Emergency Medicine, University of Florida, Gainesville, FL, USA
e-mail: Zeretzke@ufl.edu

J. Choi (✉)
Division of Pediatric Emergency Medicine, Department of Emergency Medicine, University of Florida, Gainesville, FL, USA
e-mail: joonchoi@ufl.edu

© The Author(s), under exclusive license to Springer Nature Switzerland AG 2023
C. M. Zeretzke-Bien, T. B. Swan (eds.), *Quick Hits for Pediatric Emergency Medicine*, https://doi.org/10.1007/978-3-031-32650-9_8

Modified GCS for Age < 1

Score	Motor activity	Verbal activity	Eye opening
1	None	None	None
2	Abnormal extension	Grunts or moans	To pain
3	Abnormal flexion	Cries to pain	To shout
4	Withdraws	Irritable cry	Spontaneous
5	Localizes pain	Coos and babbles	–
6	Spontaneous movement	–	–

Consider intubation for GCS < 8.

Fluid Resuscitation Guidelines

- Bolus one: 20 mL/kg normal saline (NS) (or Ringer's lactate, RL).
- Bolus two: 20 mL/kg NS or RL.
- Bolus three: 20 mL/kg NS or RL, consider starting PRBCs (uncrossmatched O-negative blood) if starting third fluid bolus in trauma patient (3:1 rule).

Fluid Maintenance Requirements

Weight (Kg) Requirements Per 24 h:

0–10 kg	100 mL/kg
10–20 kg	1000 mL for first 10 kg + 50 mL for every kg over 10 and under 20 kg
More than 20 kg	1500 mL for first 20 kg +20 mL for every kg over 20 kg

4 mL/kg/h for first 10 kg.
2 mL/kg/h for second 10 kg + 40 mL.
1 mL/kg/h for every kg >20 kg +60 mL.

Fluid Replacement for Burns

Ringer's lactate: *2–4 mL/kg/%BSA for second and third degree burns.*
   Give ½ in first 8 h and ½ in next 16 h.
   (Add maintenance fluids with 5% dextrose in children <5 years old).

Adequate Urine Output

Infant: *1 mL/kg/h.*
   Adolescent: 0.5–1 mL/kg/h.
   Estimated normal blood volume by age:

Full term = 90 mL/kg.
3–12 months = 80 mL/kg.
>1 year = 70 mL/kg.

Blood Replacement Guidelines

PRBCs: 10 mL/kg (hemoglobin rises 2–2.5 g/dL for each 10 mL/kg of RBCs transfused).
Platelets: 5–10 mL/kg should raise count by 50,000.
Fresh frozen plasma: (FFP) 10–20 mL/kg for coagulation factor replacement—raise 20%.
Factor VIII: 1 U/kg increase factor VIII plasma levels by 2%.
Factor IX: 1 U/kg increases factor IX plasma levels by 1%.

Tube Sizes (French)

	Neonate	6 months	1–2 years	5 years	8–10 years
Chest tube	10–12 F	10–12 F	16–20 F	20–28 F	28–32 F
NG tube	5–8 F	5–8 F	8–10 F	10–14 F	14–18 F
Urinary catheter	5–8 F (feeding)	8 F	8–10 F	10–12 F	12 F

General Considerations for Pediatric Trauma Patients

Size and Shape

- Greater amount of force per unit body area because of smaller body mass.
- Child's body has less fat, less elastic connective tissue, and close proximity of multiple organs, which results in high frequency of multiple organ injuries.
- Larger surface area relative to volume predisposes to thermal evaporative loss.
- Hypothermia may develop quickly and complicate hypotension.

Skeleton

- More pliable skeleton due to incomplete calcification which results in serious organ injury without overlying skeletal fracture; if rib fractures are identified, anticipate serious organ injury.
- Multiple active growth centers with unique fractures with potential growth arrest or growth abnormality.

Surface Area

- Disproportionate ratio of body surface area (highest at birth).
- Thermal energy loss is a significant stress factor in the injured child.

ABCDE of Pediatric Trauma Management

Airway and Cervical Spine Stabilization

- Establish a patent airway to provide tissue oxygenation.
- Hold cervical spine stabilization while obtaining an airway.

  - Cervical spine fractures are uncommon—more likely ligamentous injury.
  - Cervical spine fractures and injury occur higher in the C-spine due to weight of the head.
  - Flexible ligaments may allow vertebral shift and cord injury without fracture (SCIWORA).
  - *If a cervical injury is identified, there is a high chance of identifying another noncontinuous spinal injury.*
  - *Do not use NEXUS criteria under age 8 years (Fig. 8.1).*
  - *Do not use Canadian C-spine Rules under age 16 years (Fig. 8.2).*

Meets all low risk criteria?

1. No posterior midline cervical-spine tenderness.
2. No evidence of intoxication.
3. A normal level of alertness.
4. No focal neurologic deficit.
5. No painful distracting injuries.

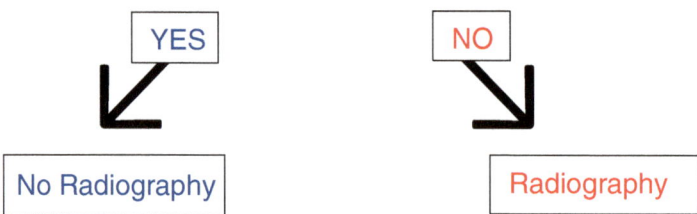

Fig. 8.1 National emergency X-radiography utilization study (NEXUS) Criteria

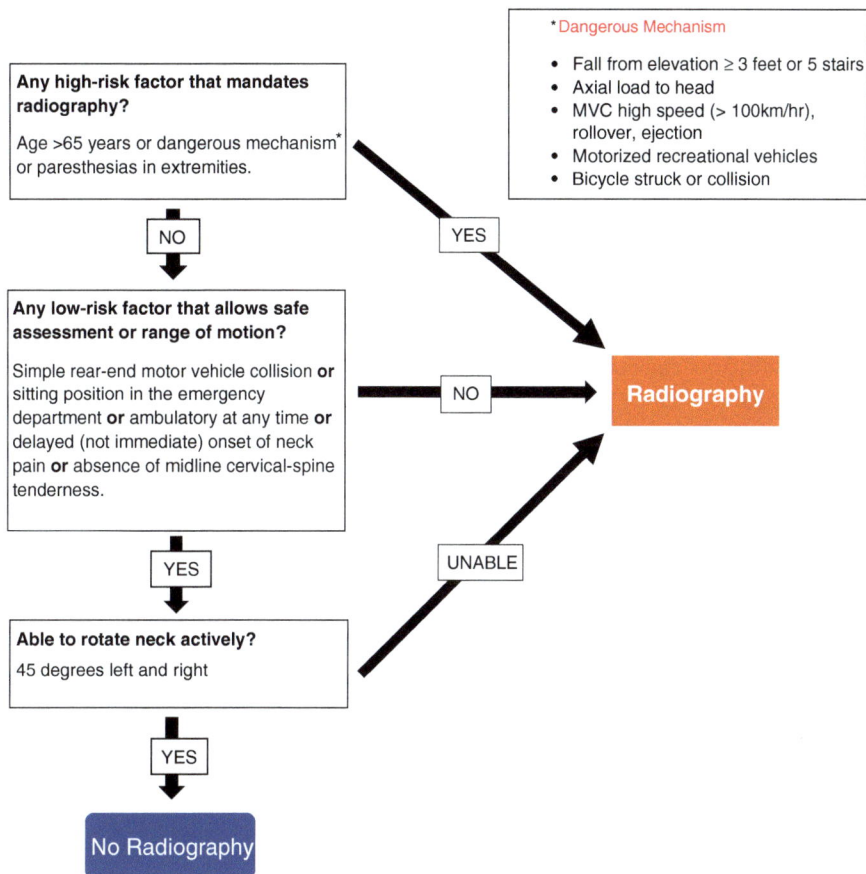

Fig. 8.2 Canadian C-spine rule

Breathing and Ventilation

- Pediatric bag mask for children <30 kg.
- Tidal volumes 4–6 mL/kg (infants and children).
- Hypoxia is the most common reason for arrest.
- With adequate perfusion and ventilation, a child should maintain a normal pH.

Circulation and Hemorrhage Control

- A child's increased physiologic reserve results in normal systolic blood pressure even in the presence of shock.

- Up to 30% of blood volume may be lost before a change in systolic blood pressure.
- Tachycardia and poor skin perfusion (cap refill) are the keys to early recognition of hypovolemia.

Disability

- Modified GCS for infants and children (see above).
- Pupil size and reactivity.
- Extremity movement and tone.
- Posturing.
- Reflexes.

Exposure

- The young child is unable to shiver.
- Thin skin and lack of subcutaneous fat.
- Larger surface area with an increased evaporative heat loss.
- Less energy reserve.
- Increased caloric expenditure.

Quick Hits Pediatric Trauma Pearls

1. Trauma is the most common cause of mortality and morbidity in the US pediatric population.
2. Accounts for >50% of all pediatric deaths.
3. Twenty thousand children die each year from injury.
4. Head injury is the leading cause of death, followed by chest and abdominal trauma.
5. Eighty-seven percent of injuries are from blunt trauma.

Chapter 9
Pediatric Head Injury Guidelines

Andrej Pogribny, Anna McFarlin, and Cristina M. Zeretzke-Bien

Abstract The pediatric head injury chapter is a poignant depiction of the widely accepted and utilized PECARN clinical decision rules for the patient in two specific age cohorts. Applying these rules can decrease the need for head CT and unnecessary radiation exposure.

Pediatric Head Injury Guidelines

- Multiple clinical decision rules have been constructed to balance minimizing unnecessary CT exposure and cost while also detecting clinically significant traumatic brain injury (ciTBIs).
- The PECARN (Pediatric Emergency Care Applied Research Network) head injury prediction rules have the highest sensitivity detecting ciTBIs, have been validated, and demonstrate reduction in both cost and utilization of head CTs.
- While the original study did not define ED observation, these authors use a timeframe of 4–6 h observation in the emergency department from time of injury.

A. Pogribny
Division of Pediatric Emergency Medicine, Children's Hospital of New Orleans, New Orleans, LA, USA

A. McFarlin (✉)
Department of Pediatrics and Division of Emergency Medicine, Louisiana State University Health Science Center, New Orleans, LA, USA

C. M. Zeretzke-Bien
Division of Pediatric Emergency Medicine, University of Florida, Gainesville, FL, USA
e-mail: Zeretzke@ufl.edu

C. M. Zeretzke-Bien, T. B. Swan (eds.), *Quick Hits for Pediatric Emergency Medicine*, https://doi.org/10.1007/978-3-031-32650-9_9

- For those in the intermediate category, one may also consider physician experience and parental preference when deciding between obtaining head CT or observing in the ED.

Pediatric Blunt Head Injury, Less Than 2 Years Old (Fig. 9.1)

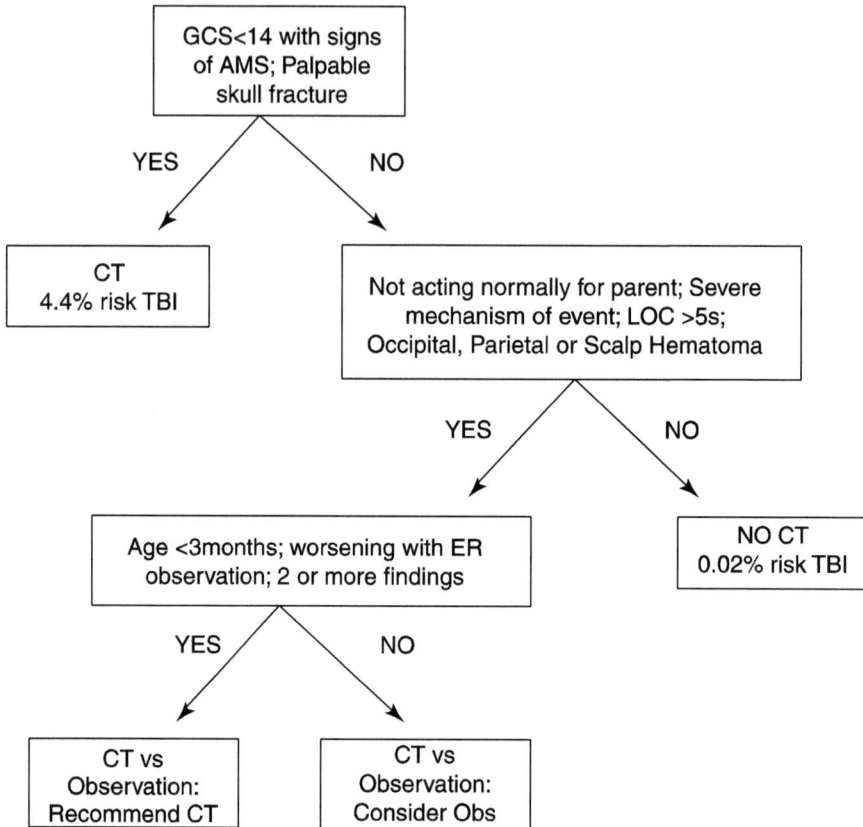

Fig. 9.1 Pediatric blunt head injury less than age 2 years old

Pediatric Blunt Head Injury, 2 Years Old and Older (Fig. 9.2)

- Definitions
  - Severe mechanism of action: Motor vehicle crash with ejection, death of a passenger, rollover, pedestrian or bicyclist struck by motor vehicle, fall from >3 ft. (<2 years old) or > 5 ft. (≥2 years old), impact by fast-moving object.
  - Altered mental status: Somnolence, agitation, slow response to external stimuli.

Reprinted with permission from Kuppermann et al. Identification of children at very low risk of clinically important brain injuries after head trauma: a prospective cohort study. *Lancet*. 2009; 374:1160–70.

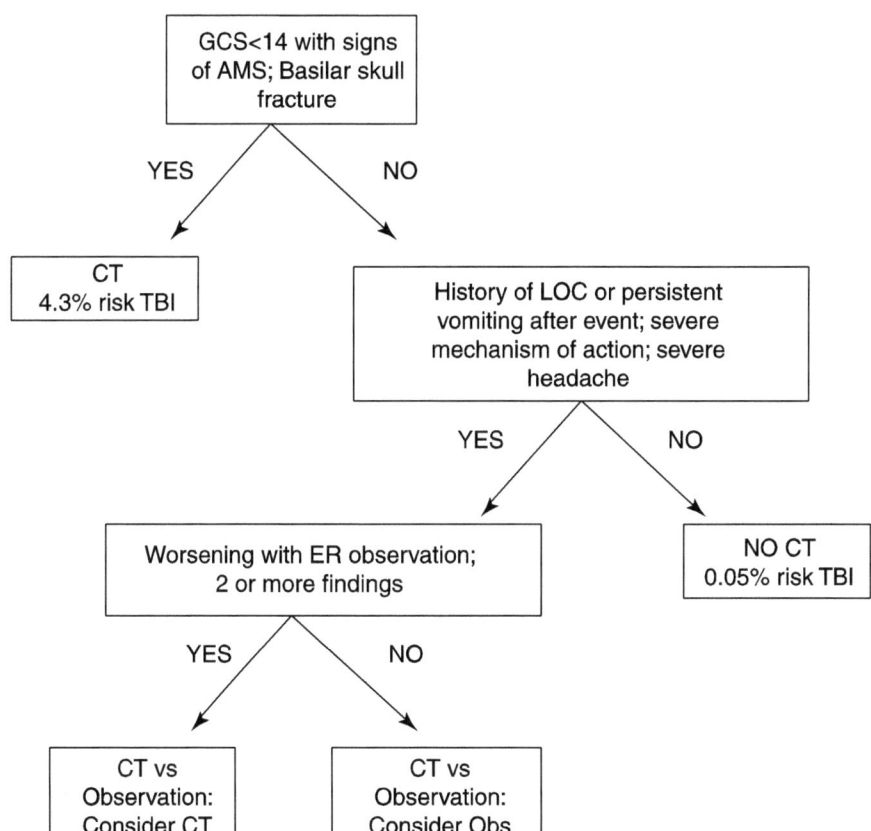

Fig. 9.2 Pediatric blunt head injury greater than age 2 years old

Chapter 10
Pediatric Burns

Elizabeth Zorovich and Cristina M. Zeretzke-Bien

Abstract Identification and classification of a burn in a pediatric patient has significant implications for care and possible transfer to a burn center. This chapter discusses characteristics of different burn classifications as well as the evidence based management required to decrease the risk of disability. A must know list of indications for admission versus transfer to a burn center is also included.

Etiology

- Often accidental but must consider nonaccidental trauma.
- Ensure reported mechanism matches pattern of burn.

Work-Up

- Ensure ABCs are intact.
- Perform primary and secondary survey.
- Ensure full exposure of the skin and remove all clothing including rings, belts, and jewelry on the body.
- Consider associated toxicities (carbon monoxide, cyanide, and hydrogen fluoride).

E. Zorovich (✉)
Pediatric Emergency Medicine, University of Florida Health Jacksonville,
Jacksonville, FL, USA
e-mail: elizabeth.zorovich@jax.ufl.edu

C. M. Zeretzke-Bien
Division of Pediatric Emergency Medicine, University of Florida, Gainesville, FL, USA
e-mail: Zeretzke@ufl.edu

C. M. Zeretzke-Bien, T. B. Swan (eds.), *Quick Hits for Pediatric Emergency
Medicine*, https://doi.org/10.1007/978-3-031-32650-9_10

Burn Classification

- First degree burn/superficial

  - Sunburn
  - Mild erythema
  - Involves epidermis only

- Second degree burn/partial thickness

  - Blisters
  - Erythematous, painful
  - Involves epidermis and dermis

- Third degree burn/full thickness

  - Waxy appearing
  - Usually insensate
  - Extending through the dermis

- Calculate body surface area (as described below) to further classify burn. Only second degree and third degree burns count towards total body surface area (TBSA).

Management

Not Severe (Examples: Superficial burns, partial thickness burns less than 10% body surface area).

- Cleanse burn with mild soap and water or dilute antiseptic solution.
- Debride wound as needed.
- Consider a topical antimicrobial: Bacitracin, neomycin, or mupirocin.
- Avoid silver sulfadiazine as it may interfere with partial thickness healing.
- Consider use of synthetic occlusive dressings.
- Ensure tetanus vaccine is updated.
- Outpatient follow-up with burn service or pediatrician depending on severity.

Severe Burns (Examples: Partial thickness burns greater than 10% body surface area, partial thickness/full thickness burns involving the face/hands/feet/cross over joints, all full thickness burns, airway involvement).

- Airway protection.
  - Place patient on oxygen.
  - Consider intubation if there are signs of inhalation injury (full thickness burns of the face or perioral region, circumferential neck burns, progressive hoarseness, soot in the nose or oral cavity).
  - Consider prophylactic intubation for patients requiring transfer to burn center with concern for altered mental status or inhalation injury.

- Fluid resuscitation.

  - Follow *Parkland Formula* using normal saline or lactated ringers.

4 mL × % BSA × weight (kg) = amount of crystalloid to be given over 24 h (mL/kg)
Give half of the amount of fluid in first 8 h, then give remaining fluids over next 16 h.

Maintenance fluids with D5NS should also be given for children under 5 years old or under 20 kg.

4 mL/kg/h for the first 10 kg of body mass,
2 mL/kg/h for the second 10 kg of body mass (11 kg–20 kg),
1 mL/kg/h for any kilogram of body mass above 20 kg.

- Urine output.

  - Place indwelling catheter.
  - Maintain urine output of 0.5–1 mL/kg/h urine in adults and 1–2 mL/kg/h in children weighing <30 kg.

- Pain control.

  - Opioids usually first line (can consider intranasal until IV established).

- Debridement.

  - Required for partial or full thickness burn.
  - Must reevaluate classification of burn after debridement.

- Antibiotics *not* indicated for prophylaxis.

  - Tetanus vaccine should be updated.

- Escharotomy burn indications.

  - Circumferential eschar involving the torso causing restricted ventilation.
  - Circumferential eschar involving extremity and causing vascular compromise.
  - Signs or symptoms of compartment syndrome or compartment pressure greater than 30 mmHg.

- Cyanide poisoning.

  - Burning of nitrogen containing polymers (plastics, wool, silk).
  - Consider treating empirically for cyanide poisoning if fire was in enclosed space.
  - First line therapy is hydroxocobalamin.

Indications for transfer to burn center and/or admission

- Partial thickness burns >10% BSA.
- Full-thickness burns of any size.
- Circumferential burn.
- Involving the face, genitals, hands, or feet.
- Electrical, high voltage, or chemical burns.
- Associated with inhalation injury.
- Burn crosses joints.
- Inability to provide adequate care for children.

Estimating Total Body Surface Area for Burns

There are three methods for estimating *total body surface area for burns* (Lund-Browder chart, Rule of 9, and the palm method). The most accurate method for pediatrics patients is the Lund-Browder chart (Figs. 10.1a, b and 10.2).

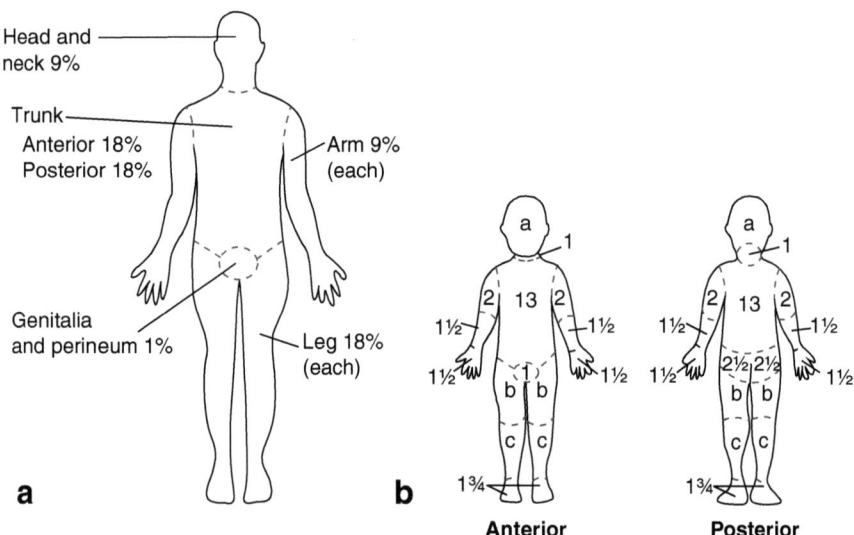

Relative percentage of body surface area (% BSA) affected by growth

	Age				
Body Part	0 yr	1 yr	5 yr	10 yr	15 yr
a = ½ of head	9 ½	8 ½	6 ½	5 ½	4 ½
b = ½ of 1 thigh	2 ¾	3 ¼	4	4 ¼	4 ½
c = ½ of 1 lower leg	2 ½	2 ½	2 ¾	3	3 ¼

Fig. 10.1 Lund-Browder chart (**a**) adult, (**b**) pediatric

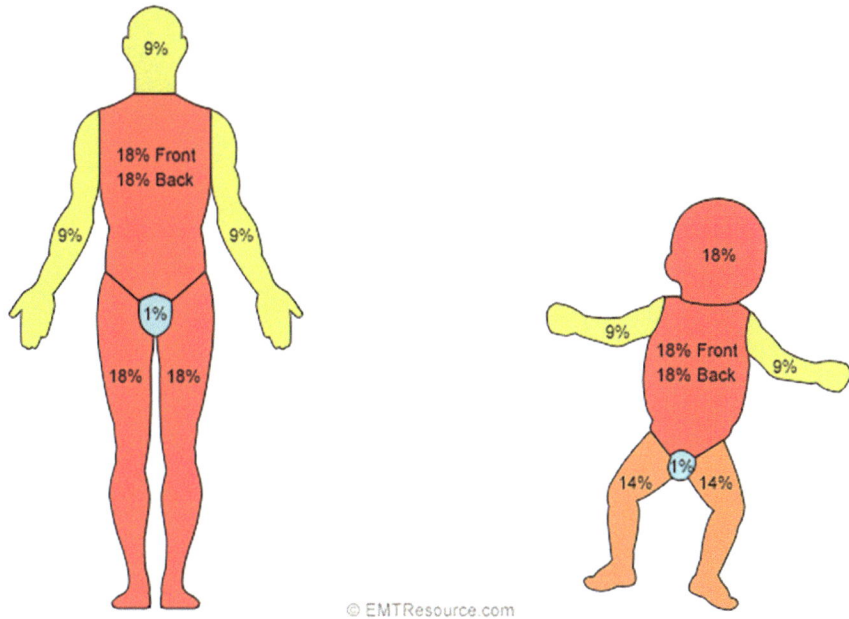

Fig. 10.2 Rules of 9

Palm method—The palm of the person who is burned, not including fingers or wrist area, is about 1% of the body surface area. Use the person's palm to measure the body surface area burned. Utilization of this method can make it hard to accurately estimate the size of a burn.

Quick Hits: Pediatric Burn Pearls

1. Always consider non-accidental trauma when evaluating a burn. Burn characteristics that should cause high suspicion for non-accidental trauma include the following: burns in varying stages of healing, sharply demarcated burn margins, uniform burn depth, no splash marks, sparing of creases or opposed skin surfaces, geometric pattern, or object imprint such as cigarette burns.
2. Consider transfer to burn center early in the evaluation.
3. Ensure proper fluid management and appropriate pain control.

Chapter 11
Procedure Pearls

Peyton Bennett, Lui Caleon, Anna McFarlin, and Cristina M. Zeretzke-Bien

Abstract This chapter is a "Quick Hit" for every common procedure that an ED provider will perform on a pediatric patient. Whether it is in an acute resuscitation requiring intubation and acquisition of intraosseous (IO) access or a laceration requiring repair to the forearm, this chapter has you covered.

Indications for Advanced Airway

- Respiratory failure as indicated by:

  - Failure to oxygenate (hypoxemia) in spite of supplemental oxygenation.
  - Failure to ventilate.
  - Clinical signs of respiratory failure include:

    Poor or absent respiratory effort.
    Poor color or cyanosis.
    Obtunded mental status.
    Pulse oximetry, end-tidal carbon dioxide (EtCO2), or partial pressure of oxygen or carbon dioxide from a blood gas can be helpful; however, intu-

P. Bennett
Pediatric Residency Program, Department of Pediatrics, Louisiana State University Health Science Center, New Orleans, LA, USA

L. Caleon
Aspen Clinic, New Orleans, LA, USA

A. McFarlin (✉)
Department of Pediatrics and Division of Emergency Medicine, Louisiana State University, New Orleans, LA, USA

C. M. Zeretzke-Bien
Division of Pediatric Emergency Medicine, University of Florida, Gainesville, FL, USA
e-mail: Zeretzke@ufl.edu

C. M. Zeretzke-Bien, T. B. Swan (eds.), *Quick Hits for Pediatric Emergency Medicine*, https://doi.org/10.1007/978-3-031-32650-9_11

bation should not be delayed in patient with clinical evidence of respiratory failure in order to obtain such measurements.

– Inability to protect airway:

Decreased level of consciousness (GCS < 8).
Airway obstruction (examples include angioedema, retropharyngeal abscess, epiglottitis, smoke inhalation, neck hematoma).

Airway Adjuncts

Nasopharyngeal Airway "Nasal Trumpet" (Fig. 11.1)

- *Sizing*: Measure from patient's nare to their tragus.
- *Insertion*: Lubricate device and insert with bevel towards the nasal septum. Once in place, the tip should be visible posterior to uvula.

Oropharyngeal Airway (Fig. 11.2)

- Indicated in unconscious patients to prevent airway occlusion from a collapsing tongue.
- *Sizing*: Measure from the corner of the mouth to angle of mandible.
- *Insertion*: Use tongue blade to depress the tongue as you insert the airway with tip pointed to the floor of the mouth.

Fig. 11.1 Nasopharyngeal airway "nasal trumpet"

Fig. 11.2 Oropharyngeal airway

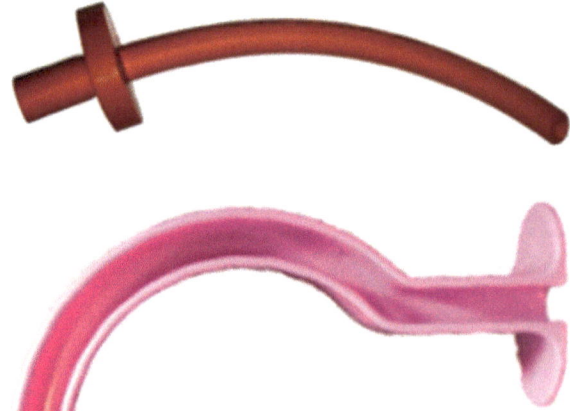

Laryngoscope Blades

Miller blades		Macintosh blades	
00	Small premature	1	Term infant*
0	Premature	2	Child (2–9 years)
1	Term infant	3	Medium adult
2	Child (2–9 years)	4	Large adult
3	Medium adult		
4	Large adult		
Pros: Takes up less space in the mouth, designed to lift the epiglottis directly		*Pros*: Designed to sweep and contain the tongue	

*not preferred in this age group

Video laryngoscopy has become increasingly popular for first attempt at intubation providing indirect visualization of the airway. Blade and monitor types are brand specific and appropriate training should be provided to ensure proficiency with the available equipment at an institution.

Endotracheal Tubes (Fig. 11.3)

Sizing

- Equation: $\dfrac{Age + 4}{4}$
- Use ½ size smaller for cuffed tube. Cuffed tubes generally preferred in all but neonates.

Depth

- Equation: $3 \times ETT$ size.
- Measure at the teeth since the lips can swell.

Confirmation

- CXR: Between clavicles and carina, by 1st/2nd ribs.
- Continuous end-tidal CO_2 or colorimetry.
- US: At sternal notch.
- Auscultation.
- Direct visualization.

Fig. 11.3 Endotracheal
tubes

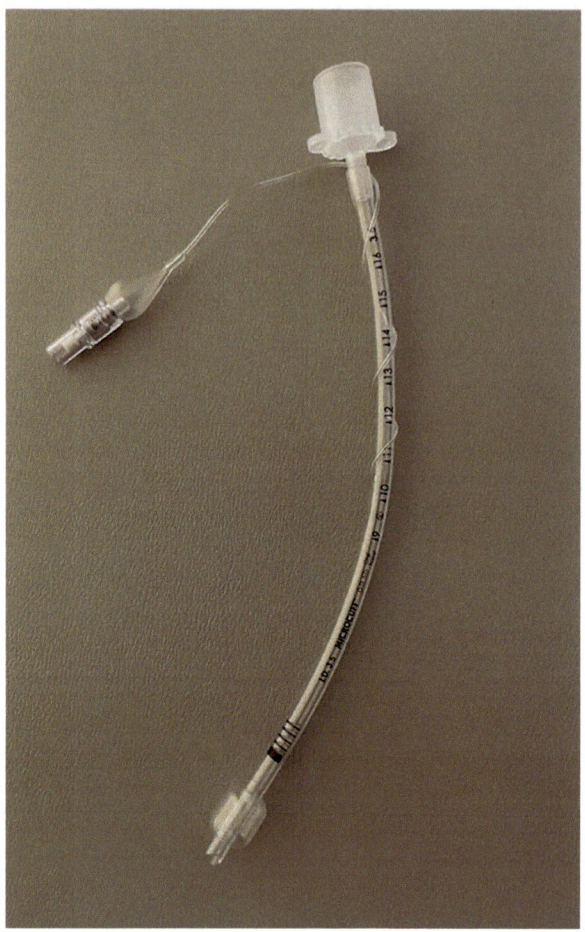

Laryngeal Mask Airways

LMAs are supraglottic airway devices which may be used in the event of a difficult
or failed airway. LMAs are typically very effective for ventilation but do not provide
protection against aspiration.

Weight (kg)	Mask size	Max cuff volume (mL)
<5	1	4
5–10	1.5	7
10–20	2	10
20–30	2.5	14
30–50	3	20
50–70	4	30
70–100	5	40
100+	6	50

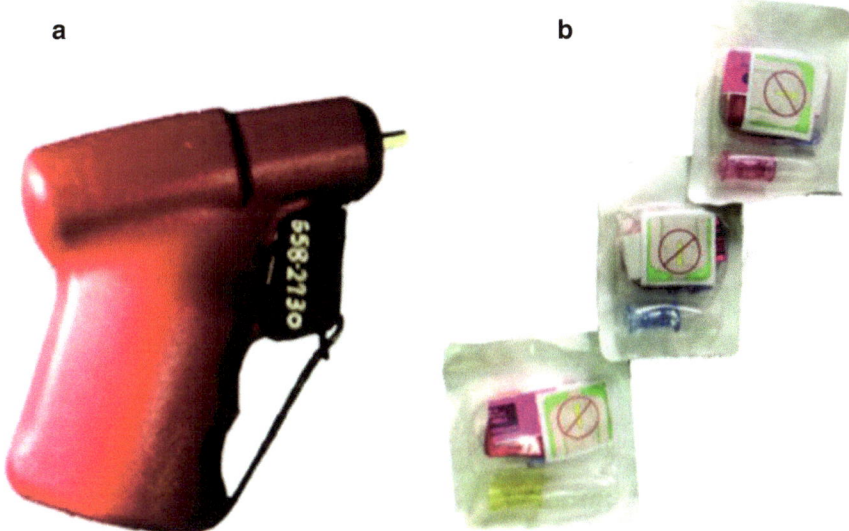

Fig. 11.4 (**a**) Drill and (**b**) drill bits for intraosseous access

Intraosseous Access

Indications

- Failure to gain peripheral venous access after approximately 90 s or two peripheral IV attempts in a critically ill patient.
- Manual or battery-operated drill style insertion options (Fig. 11.4).

Contraindications

- Overlying skin/tissue infection or burn.
- Fractured target bone.
- Prior attempt or previous IO in same bone in last 24–48 h.
- History of osteogenesis imperfecta, osteoporosis, or osteopetrosis.

Most Common Pediatric Sites

- *Proximal tibia*: Two finger breadths below the patella, medial to the tibial tuberosity.
- *Distal tibia*: 3 cm proximal to medial malleolus on the flat central aspect of tibia.
- *Distal femur*: 3 cm proximal to femoral condyle on anterolateral surface.

Quick Hits IO Access Pearls

1. Aspirate bone marrow and flush with 20 mL to ensure placement and patency.

   (a) Aspiration may not always produce blood even with a properly placed IO needle.
   (b) Penetration past the posterior tibial cortex is a common pitfall in small children. Go slow and assess posteriorly for signs of extravasation.

2. Instill lidocaine (max 3 mg/kg) to minimize discomfort prior to using for conscious patients.

External Jugular Vein Cannulation

Contraindications

- Not recommended for use for high-pressure IV contrast agent.

Procedure

- Place patient in Trendelenburg position to fill the external jugular vein.
- Rotate the head to the opposite side and have an assistant stabilize the head.
- Clean site.
- Lightly compress the vein with a free finger above the clavicle to engorge the vein and apply traction to skin.
- Ultrasound assistance or guidance may assist in location.
- Puncture midway between the angle of the jaw and midclavicular line aiming toward the ipsilateral shoulder.
- Once flash is obtained, decrease insertion angle and advance catheter.
- Verify ability to draw back and flush, and secure with tape/dressing.

Lumbar Puncture

Indications

- To obtain cerebrospinal fluid for analysis.
- To determine opening pressure or therapeutically reduce intracranial pressure.

Contraindications

- Overlying skin/tissue infection.
- Presence of increased intracranial pressure caused by space-occupying lesion.
- Coagulopathy.
- Severe thrombocytopenia.

Procedure

- Plan for pain control: Local anesthesia (topical and/or injected); sucrose orally for infants.
- Consider some degree of sedation depending on patient's age and clinical status.
- Follow sterile precautions.
- Have an assistant place patient with knees and hips flexed toward the chest to increase inter-disc spacing. Position may be achieved in lateral decubitus or seated positions in all ages. Severe neck flexion has not been shown to facilitate the procedure and may cause apnea in infants.
- Identify the L4 vertebra by palpating the left and right superior iliac crests; make a superficial mark with marker or indentation with a pen cap or your fingernail in the interspace just above or below L4.
- Direct needle toward patient's umbilicus.
- Withdraw stylet to assess for CSF flow.
- Use fluid collected for opening pressure in manometer for tube #1.
- Normal opening pressure = 12–20. For accurate assessment of opening pressure, patient must be in lateral recumbent position.

Lab Orders

- *Tube 1*: gram stain, culture, and sensitivities.
- *Tube 2*: protein and glucose.
- *Tube 3*: cell count and differential.
- *Tube 4*: Hold and consider HSV studies (especially if CSF bloody).

Incision and Drainage

Indications

- Localized abscess/fluid collections.

Procedure

- Ultrasound can be used to differentiate fluid collections from localized tissue inflammation. Look for hypoechoic areas suggestive of abscess versus diffuse "cobblestoning" seen with cellulitis.
- Analgesia.

  - *Topical*: EMLA/LMX for closed lesions, LET for open lesions.
  - *Local*: Lidocaine intradermal.

- Make sure to make an incision approximately 2/3 the size of the pocket to ensure adequate drainage and to prevent fluid accumulation.
- Probe the wound and dissect the wound to break open loculations.
- There is no proven benefit to routine packing of cutaneous abscesses as it does not appear to prevent recurrence.
- Consider the alternative loop drain technique to prevent large incisions and to encourage continued drainage.
- Loop ties can be fashioned from Penrose drains or from the edge of a sterile glove.

Laceration Repair (Fig. 11.5)

Wound Approximation Options

Sutures

Nonabsorbable sutures	Absorbable sutures	Tensile strength
Silk	Fast absorbing plain gut	5–7 days
Nylon (Ethilon)	Cat/chromic gut	2–3 weeks
Polypropylene (Prolene)	Poliglecaprone (Monocryl)	2 weeks
	Vicryl rapide	2 weeks
	Polydioxanone (PDS)	50% at 4 weeks
	Polyglactin (Vicryl)	25% at 4 weeks
	Less strength but does not require removal	

- Gauge increases resulting in a finer/thinner suture.
- Gauge roughly estimates number of knot throws needed (Figs. 11.6 and 11.7).

Lacerations: Overview for Repair

- *Assess*

  - Size, if more complex, consider consultation.
  - Foreign body?
  - Neurovascularly intact?
  - Infection risk (tetanus, rabies, grossly contaminated wound).

Laceration Repair

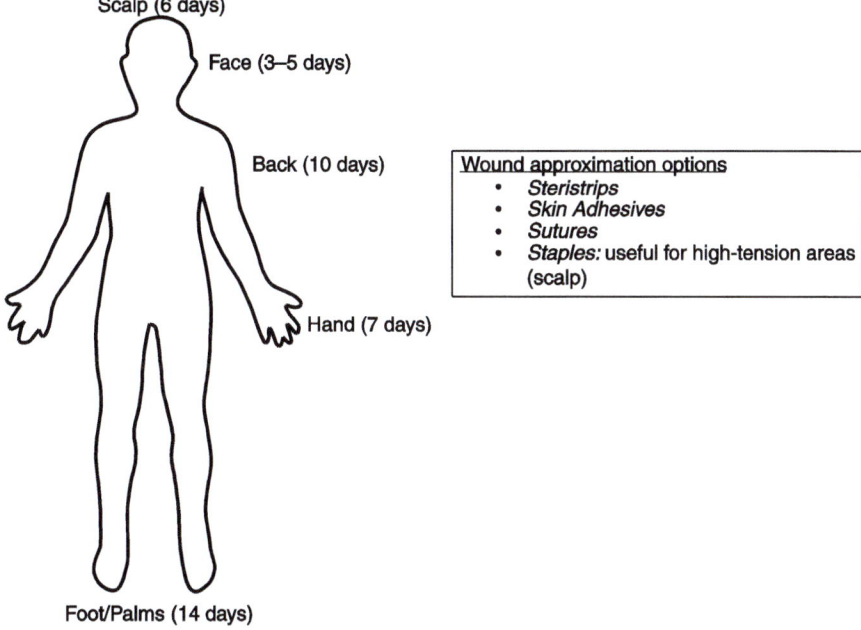

Fig. 11.5 Approximate time ranges for wound healing/suture removal

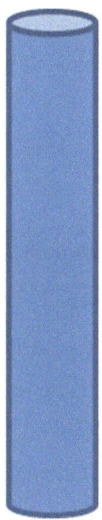

Fig. 11.6 Suture gauge 2.0

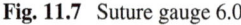

Fig. 11.7 Suture gauge 6.0

- *Anesthesia*
  - Child life.
  - Midazolam 0.5 mg/kg PO or intranasally (max 1 mL to each nare).
  - 1% intradermal lidocaine.

      with epi (max = 0.7 cc/kg).
      without epi (max = 0.4 cc/kg).

- *Topical*
  - LET (4% lidocaine, 1:2000 epi, 0.5% tetracaine).
  - Max = 7 mg lidocaine/kg (0.2 cc/kg).
  - Fill wound and top with saturated gauze or cotton ball, hold in place with adhesive dressing; leave for at least 20–30 min.
  - Duration, 45–60 min.

- *Irrigation:* sterile saline or water.
- *Suturing*
  - Deep sutures: absorbable monofilament.

  (usually Vicryl®, PDS, chromic gut).

  - Superficial sutures: nonabsorbable monofilament.

  (usually Prolene®, Ethilon®) *or* absorbable sutures such as fast absorbing plain gut or Vicryl® Rapide.

- *Dressing:* leave in place for 24 h, and then clean twice daily with clean water and mild soap.
  - Steri-Strips.
  - Bacitracin.
  - Sterile gauze.

• *Suture removal: see chart.*

Location	Anesthetic	Deep suture	Superficial suture	Dressing	Suture removal	Special
Scalp	1% lido w/epi	3–0/4–0 Vicryl	Staples preferred. If suturing, 5–0/4–0 nonabsorbable suture, fast absorbing plain gut	Bacitracin, air	5–7 days	Pressure dressing if early hematoma
Pinna (ear)	1% lido	5–0 Vicryl in perichondrium	6–0 nonabsorbable suture, fast absorbing plain gut	Bacitracin, light pressure dressing	5 days	
Eyelid/ eyebrow	1% lido	5–0 Vicryl	6–0/5–0 nonabsorbable suture, fast absorbing plain gut	Bacitracin, air	4–5 days	Do not shave hair
Lip	1% lido w/epi	5–0 Vicryl	6–0 nonabsorbable suture (rapid)	Air		If through the vermillion border, consider plastics
Face Forehead	1% lido w/epi	5–0 Vicryl	6–0 nonabsorbable suture, fast absorbing plain gut	Bacitracin, air	4–6 days	Facial nerve—Ensure it is in tact
Neck	1% lido w/epi	4–0 Vicryl	5–0 nonabsorbable suture		4–6 days	Thru platysma, needs consult
Trunk	1% lido w/epi	4–0 Vicryl	5–0/4–0 nonabsorbable suture	Bacitracin	7–10 days	r/o deeper path, may need consult
Extremities/ buttocks	1% lido w/epi	4–0 Vicryl 5–0 Vicryl	4–0 nonabsorbable suture, 3–0 for over joints 5–0/6–0 nonabsorbable suture (rapid)		7–10 days 10–14 days if over joint	Check if neurovascularly intact
Hands	1% lido	None	5–0/6–0 nonabsorbable suture 5–0 rapid if <5 y.o.		7–10 days 10–14 days if over joint	
Nail beds	1% lido	None	6–0 Vicryl	Bacitracin/splint/ Xeroform gauze		If amputation, splint+ antibiotics
Feet/sole	1% lido	None	5–0/4–0/3–0 nonabsorbable suture	Bacitracin, Xeroform	10–14 days	Kling wrap
Scrotum	1% lido	None	5–0/6–0 Vicryl or 5–0 gut	Bacitracin, air, 4 × 4, fluff, scrotal support		Consider specialty consult
Penis	1% lido		5–0 nonabsorbable suture		6–8 days	Consider specialty consult

Chapter 12
Pediatric Orthopedics

Tricia B. Swan and Yiraima Medina-Blasini

Abstract This chapter is packed with great "Quick Hits" about "not to be missed" pediatric orthopedic injuries and disorders. It starts with unique fracture patterns and the mnemonic for elbow ossification centers and continues through the suggested management of specific fractures. This chapter also includes some of the most common orthopedic issues in children including common apophysitis presentations, septic arthritis, and the limping child. The pearls at the end of the chapter are a must-read.

Pediatric Specific Fracture Patterns

- Greenstick Fracture.

  - Incomplete fracture in which one cortex remains intact.
  - These fractures might require closed reduction to avoid abnormal growth.

- Torus Fracture.

  - Common in young children.
  - Bone cortex buckles usually at the metaphysis–diaphysis junction.

T. B. Swan (✉)
Division of Pediatric Emergency Medicine, University of Florida, Gainesville, FL, USA
e-mail: tfalgiani@ufl.edu

Y. Medina-Blasini
Division of Pediatric Emergency Medicine, Department of Emergency Medicine, HCA Florida Kendall Hospital, Miami, FL, USA

C. M. Zeretzke-Bien, T. B. Swan (eds.), *Quick Hits for Pediatric Emergency Medicine*, https://doi.org/10.1007/978-3-031-32650-9_12

- Bowing Fracture.

    - Plastic (bowing) deformity.
    - Orthopedic referral: obvious forearm deformity or restricted pronation and/or supination.

- Salter Harris Fractures (SALTR) (Fig. 12.1).

    - Type I: Fracture through the physis without injury to epiphysis or metaphysis.
    - Type II: Fracture through the physis and extends through metaphysis (most common).
    - Type III: Fracture through the physis and extends through epiphysis.
    - Type IV: Fracture traverses through epiphysis, physis, and metaphysis.
    - Type V: Crush injury of physis (very rare and has the worst prognosis).

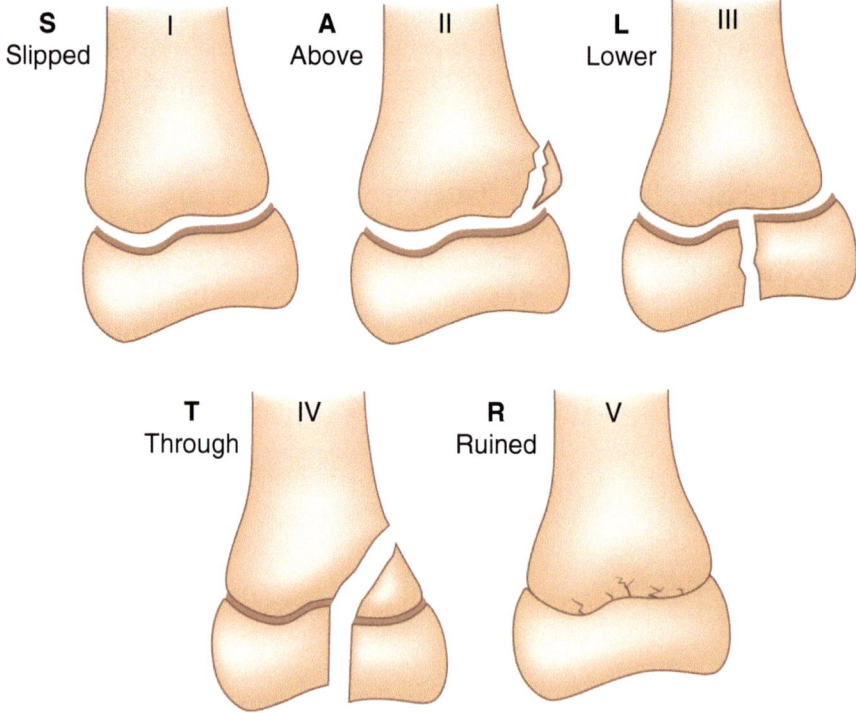

Fig. 12.1 Salter Harris fractures

Pediatric Elbow Ossification Centers (CRITOE) (Fig. 12.2)

Supracondylar Fractures of the Humerus

- 50% of all fractures of the elbow.
- Extension type fracture.

  - Most common (95%).
  - Distal fragment displaced posteriorly.
  - Occurs from fall onto outstretched hand (FOOSH).

- Flexion type fracture.

  - Rare.
  - Distal fragment displaced anteriorly.
  - Occurs from falling directly onto flexed elbow.

- Plain AP and lateral X-rays should be obtained.
- Posterior fat pad sign on lateral view is always pathologic and should raise suspicion of occult elbow fracture, even if not evident on plain film.

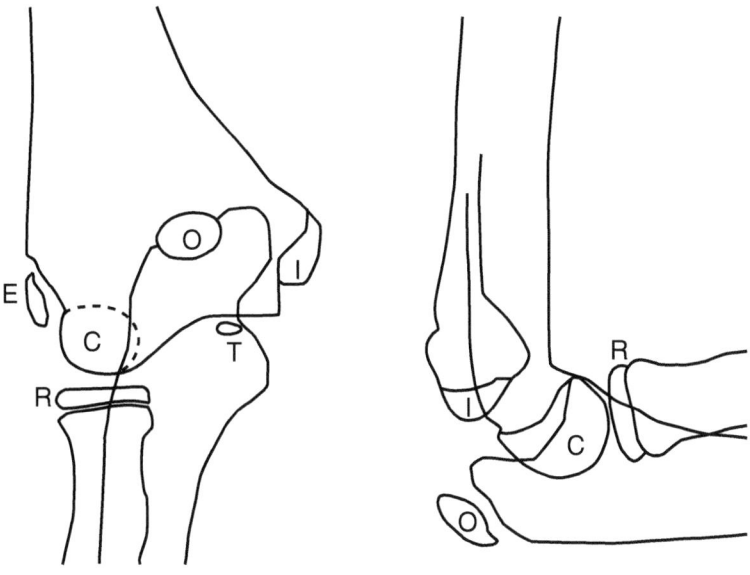

C – capitellum	(1–2 years)	T – trochlear	(6–8 years)
R – radial head	(2–4 years)	O – olecronon	(8–10 years)
I – internal malleous	(4–6 years)	E – external malleolus	(10–12 years)

Fig. 12.2 Pediatric Elbow Ossification Center (CRITOE)

- Neurovascular status of the arm and hand must be assessed immediately.
- *Management.*

  - Pain control.
  - Posterior long arm splint.
  - Non-displaced type I supracondylar fracture: Urgent orthopedic follow-up as outpatient.
  - Displaced type II and type III supracondylar fracture: Emergent orthopedic consultation (may require transfer to another facility).

- Appropriate and timely treatment of supracondylar fractures has 2 goals:

  - Avoid neurologic and vascular issues.
  - Prevent long term angular and extension deformities (Figs. 12.3 and 12.4).

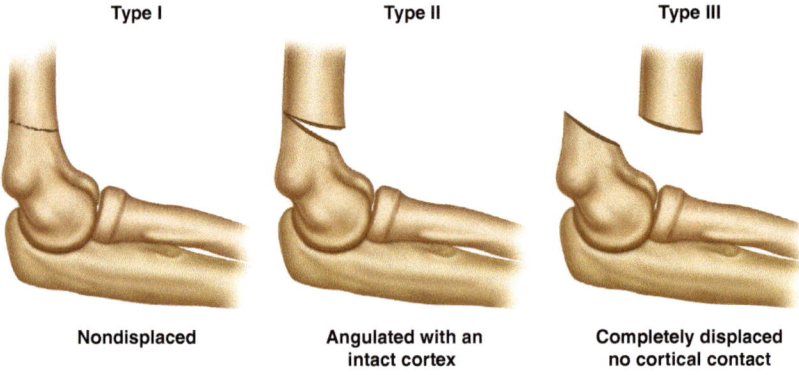

Figs. 12.3 Gartland classification of supracondylar humerus fractures

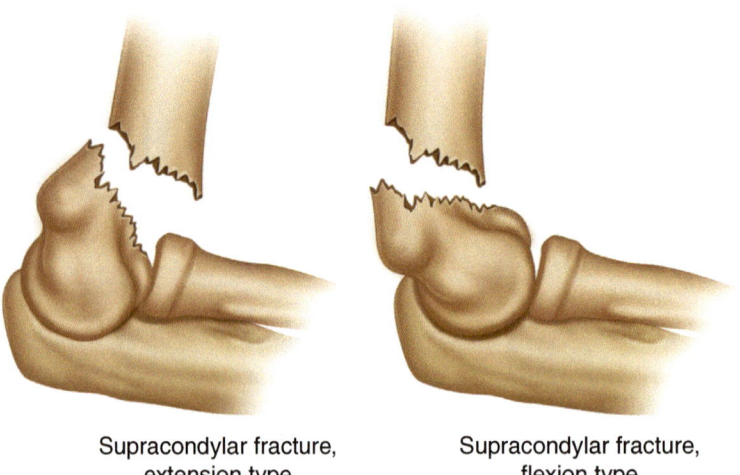

Figs. 12.4 Extension and flexion types of supracondylar humerus fractures

Neurovascular Injuries in Supracondylar Fractures

Neurovascular structure	Finding
Anterior interosseous nerve	Most common nerve injury Unable to do OK sign with finger and thumb Unable to bend the tip of the index finger
Radial nerve	Second most common nerve injury Weakness or inability to extend wrist or fingers Unable to give "thumbs up" sign Loss of sensation in first web space
Ulnar nerve	Unable to abduct digits 3–5 (spread fingers) Loss of sensation in the pinky finger
Median nerve	Unable to flex digits 2–3 Unable to grasp object or finger Loss of sensation on volar aspect of index finger
Brachial artery	Absent radial pulse Cold, pale, pulseless hand

Common Pediatric Fractures and Management

Fracture	X-Ray	ED management	Immobilization
Clavicle	AP, cranial/caudal tilt view	Outpatient follow up unless fracture is open or there is skin tenting, neurovascular injury, significant degree of angulation or displacement >2 cm in an older child	Arm sling (recommended) or figure of 8 wrap (1–4 weeks) Orthopedic follow-up for children who participate in athletics otherwise can follow up with their pediatrician
Elbow supracondylar type I	AP in extension, lateral with 90° of flexion, oblique	Outpatient follow-up in 3–5 days	Posterior long arm splint with elbow in 90° of flexion with forearm in neutral position Be sure not to flex arm more than 90° to avoid vascular compromise and compartment syndrome*
Elbow supracondylar types II and III	AP in extension, lateral with 90° of flexion, oblique	Emergent orthopedic consultation; closed or open reduction	Long arm immobilization while awaiting orthopedic consult

Fracture	X-Ray	ED management	Immobilization
Elbow lateral condyle	AP in extension, lateral with 90° of flexion, oblique	Emergent orthopedic consultation; surgical repair	Long arm immobilization while awaiting orthopedic consult
Distal radius/ulna fracture	Wrist AP, lateral (+/− forearm and elbow X-rays)	Outpatient follow-up unless fracture is open, neurovascular injury, significant displacement, or degree of angulation >10° (>6 years of age) or > 15° (<6 years of age)	Volar splint with arm sling Orthopedic follow-up in 1 week
Night stick (midshaft ulnar fracture)	Forearm AP, lateral (+/− elbow X-rays)	Outpatient follow-up unless fracture is open, neurovascular injury, significant displacement, or degree of angulation >10° (>6 years of age) or > 15° (<6 years of age)	Posterior long arm splint Orthopedic follow-up in 1 week
Monteggia (ulnar fracture with radial head dislocation)	Forearm AP, lateral Elbow AP, lateral	Orthopedics consult Closed or open reduction	Long arm immobilization while awaiting orthopedic consult
Galeazzi (radial shaft fracture with disruption of the radioulnar joint)	Forearm AP, lateral Elbow AP, lateral	Orthopedics consult Closed or open reduction	Long arm immobilization while awaiting orthopedic consult
Colles (distal radius fracture with dorsal displacement and volar angulation)	Forearm AP, lateral Elbow AP, lateral +/− wrist	Outpatient follow-up unless fracture is open, neurovascular injury, rotational deformity or degree of angulation >40°, or severe displacement; if not appropriate for outpatient follow-up, orthopedic consultation for closed or open reduction	Long arm posterior or sugar tong splint Orthopedic follow-up in 3–5 days If orthopedic consultation is required, long arm immobilization while awaiting orthopedic consult
Smith (distal radius fracture with volar displacement and dorsal angulation)	Forearm AP, lateral Elbow AP, lateral +/− wrist	Outpatient follow-up unless fracture is open, neurovascular injury, rotational deformity or degree of angulation >10°, or severe displacement; if not appropriate for outpatient follow-up, orthopedic consultation for closed or open reduction	Long arm posterior or sugar tong splint Orthopedic follow-up in 3–5 days If orthopedic consultation is required, long arm immobilization while awaiting orthopedic consult
Buckle (AKA torus fracture)	Wrist AP, lateral, oblique Forearm AP, lateral	Outpatient follow-up unless fracture is open or neurovascular injury	Short arm cast or removable Velcro wrist splint Orthopedic follow-up in 1–2 weeks

Fracture	X-Ray	ED management	Immobilization
Toddler fracture (spiral tibial shaft fracture)	Tibia and fibula AP, lateral, oblique	Outpatient follow-up unless fracture is open or neurovascular injury	Long leg posterior splint; orthopedic follow-up in 3–5 days
Femoral shaft	Femur AP, lateral Pelvis X-ray Knee AP, lateral	Emergent orthopedic consultation	Immobilization while awaiting orthopedic consult Consider traction techniques
Ankle triplane (complex tibial physis fracture occurring in 3 planes)	Ankle AP, lateral, mortise CT scan of ankle	Emergent orthopedic consultation	Short or long leg immobilization with ankle stirrups while awaiting orthopedic consult
Tillaux ankle Fracture (salter Harris III type fracture of the distal tibia)	Ankle AP, lateral, mortise CT scan of ankle	Emergent orthopedic consultation	Short or long leg immobilization with ankle stirrups while awaiting orthopedic consult

Common Splints and Indications

Splint	Indication
Thumb spica	Scaphoid and lunate fractures, thumb fracture, non-displaced first metacarpal fracture
Radial gutter	Non-rotated/non-displaced second and third metacarpal or proximal and middle phalangeal fractures
Ulnar gutter	Non-rotated/non-displaced fourth and fifth metacarpal or proximal and middle phalangeal fractures
Dorsal/volar	Carpal bone fractures (except for trapezium or scaphoid fractures), distal radius buckle fracture, soft tissue injury to hand and wrist
Sugar tong	Distal radius and ulna fractures
Double sugar tong	Unstable forearm and/or elbow fractures
Long arm posterior	Proximal and midshaft radius and ulna fractures, non-buckle type distal radius fractures, distal humerus fractures
Buddy taping	Non-angulated/non-displaced fractures of the phalanx
Aluminum U-shaped finger	Non-angulated/non-displaced fractures of the phalanx
Knee immobilizer	Knee soft tissue injuries, post-reduction of patella dislocations
Long leg posterior	Proximal tibia and fibula fractures, knee soft tissue injuries and patellar fractures, distal femur or femoral shaft fractures that do not require traction splint
Short leg posterior	Non-displaced malleolar fractures, midshaft and distal tibia and fibula fracture, severe ankle sprains, tarsal and metatarsal fractures (make sure to extend splint past toes)

Splint	Indication
Short leg posterior with ankle stirrup	Reduced ankle dislocation +/− fracture, unstable ankle fracture
Ankle stirrup	Non-displaced malleolar fractures, severe ankle sprains
High top walking boot	Non-displaced distal tibia and fibula fractures, severe ankle sprains, tarsal and metatarsal fractures
Hard sole shoe	Non-displaced, non-angulated metatarsal fracture, phalanx (toe) fracture

Splinting Complications

Contact dermatitis/skin irritation	
Pressure injuries/ulceration	
Loss of fracture reduction	
Compartment syndrome (rare, 6 P's):	Pain out of proportion (earliest sign) Paresthesia Paralysis Pallor Poikilothermia Pulselessness (late sign)

Nursemaid's Elbow

- Radial head subluxation or annular ligament displacement.
- Age presentation: 6 months–5 years old (peak age: 2–3 years old).
- Classic mechanism: Arm traction/pulling (can occur by other mechanisms).
- Clinical presentation:

  - Child refuses to move the arm and holds the arm slightly flexed at the elbow and pronated.
- Management:

  - Closed reduction technique:

       Hyperpronation (higher success rate).
       Supination-flexion.
       Should see immediate use of the arm after reduction.

- Elbow X-ray is indicated for those cases where the mechanism or clinical presentation is atypical or reduction maneuvers are unsuccessful.

The Limping Child

- Limping can be due to pain, deformity, infection, or weakness.
- The differential diagnosis is broad and ranges from minor to life-threatening causes.

Differential diagnosis (mnemonic: STOP LIMPING)
Septic arthritis
Toddler's fracture
Osteomyelitis
Perthes' disease
Limb leg discrepancy
Irritable hip
Malignancy
Pyomyositis or myositis
Iliopsoas abscess
Neurologic
Gastrointestinal/genitourinary

Septic Arthritis

- 90% of cases: lower extremity (knee and hip).
- >90% of cases involve a single joint.
- Most common bacteria: S. aureus.
- Clinical presentation: swelling, joint pain, fever, limp or refusal to bear weight, pseudoparalysis, pain with passive or active range of motion.

    - Fever can be absent in 1/3 of the cases.
    - Extremity position: abduction and externally rotated.

- Kocher criteria (only applies to septic arthritis of the HIP joint):

Non-weight bearing	Probability of septic arthritis of the hip:
Temp >38.5 °C/101.3 °F	1 of 4 criteria present = 3%
ESR > 40 mm/h	2 of 4 criteria present = 40%
WBC > 12,000 cells/mm^3	3 of 4 criteria present = 93%
	4 of 4 criteria present = 99%

- Evaluation:

    - CBC, ESR, CRP, blood culture, synovial fluid WBC count, gram stain and culture.

        WBC (synovial fluid) > 50,000 cells/mm^3 indicates septic arthritis.

    - X-rays: to exclude other conditions.
    - Ultrasound: joint effusion may be present.
    - MRI: most sensitive but might not be readily available in the ED or may require sedation of patient to obtain.

- Management.

    - Pain control.

- – Empiric IV antibiotics: Clindamycin, +/– Vancomycin. Add Rocephin for sexually active adolescent or ill appearing children.
- – Emergent orthopedic consultation for surgical intervention.

Transient Synovitis of the Hip

- Associated with recent viral infections.
- Age presentation: 3–8 years old.
- Bilateral involvement in 5% cases.
- Diagnosis of exclusion.
- Management: Pain control with NSAIDs.

Legg-Calve-Perthes Disease

- Idiopathic avascular necrosis of the femoral head.
- Age presentation: 3–12 years old (peak age 5–9 years old); more common in males.
- 10–20% cases are bilateral.
- Pelvis X-ray (AP and frog view).
- Management: Non-weight bearing and pediatric orthopedic consultation.

Slipped Capital Femoral Epiphysis (SCFE)

- Slip of the femoral epiphysis medially.
- Risk factor: obesity.
- Clinical presentation: hip pain or referred thigh and knee pain, altered gait.
- Pelvis X-ray (AP and frog view): "ice cream cone sign".
- Management:
  - – Non-weight bearing.
  - – Orthopedic consult for operative management.
  - – Complications: Avascular necrosis, chondrolysis, femoroacetabular impingement.

Apophysitis

- Overuse syndrome.
- Stress injury or inflammation of the apophysis.
  - – Apophysis: growth plate area where a tendon or ligament attaches.

Disorder	Clinical presentation	Possible X-ray findings	Management
Little leaguer/pitcher elbow	Medial epicondylitis More common in boys; 9–12 y/o Tenderness over medial epicondyle Elbow pain that worsens with throwing Extension of the elbow can be limited	Non-specific Irregular or widened medial epicondylar physis	Rest/stop activity Ice Anti-inflammatory medications/NSAIDs Stretching and/or strengthening exercises Physical therapy
Osgood Schlatter's disease	Jumping or running athletes Boys > girls 25% cases are bilateral Tenderness at the tibial tubercle Pain increases with squatting, climbing stairs, jumping, or forced knee extension	Normal Fragmentation of the tibial tubercle	
Siding-Larsen-Johansson	Tenderness over inferior pole of the patella	Normal Fragmentation or small avulsion at inferior pole of the patella	
Sever's disease	Common in runners, soccer players, and jumping athletes Heel pain Tenderness at the insertion of the Achilles' tendon on the calcaneus	Usually normal Widening of the growth plate	

Quick Hit Orthopedic Pearls

1. Any neurovascular injury/deficit, compartment syndrome, open or multiple fractures should be evaluated by an orthopedic specialist in the emergency department.
2. If orthopedic consultation should be required or you are transferring the patient for further management, the patient should be made NPO.
3. Children with suspected fractures or obvious deformity should have expedited pain control.
4. Consider radiographic imagining of the joint above and the joint below the suspected fracture site.
5. Splinting of the joint above and joint below will provide optimal comfort while decreasing the likelihood of additional injury.
6. Splints are often the initial choice of management for fractures to allow for swelling and decrease the risk of compartment syndrome.
7. Assess neurovascular status of the involved extremity before and after a splint is placed.

8. Non-accidental trauma should be in your differential for all children with fractures. Highly suspicious fracture patterns for abuse include: posterior rib fractures, metaphyseal bucket handle/corner fractures, fractures in non-ambulatory
   patients, bilateral long bone fractures, complex skull fractures and spinous process fractures.
9. In cases where apophysitis is highly suspected, X-rays should be ordered to
   evaluate for avulsion fracture.

Chapter 13
Pediatric Altered Mental Status

Tricia B. Swan and Amit Patel

Abstract A quick chapter on the approach to pediatric altered mental status. The mnemonic AEIOU TIPS is a comprehensive heuristic to work through the possible etiology of the patient's altered state. The chapter also includes some empiric bedside therapies for potentially reversible causes as well as some pearls to remember in all cases.

Altered mental status in children can be extremely subtle. Looking for age specific behaviors can help. This can range from being awake and alert with slight irritability to a child who is truly somnolent and lethargic.

When thinking of children with altered mental status a broad differential needs to be kept. The biggest enemy can be anchoring bias.

Much information can be obtained by just the general appearance of a child. These salient features can be categorized by the mnemonic *TICLS*.

Category	Feature
Tone	Spontaneous movements of extremities/torso/head, active vs. listless
Interaction	Alert/engaged, playing, smiling, reaches, interacts
Consolable	Consolable by caregiver, appropriate for situation
Look/gaze	Fixed gaze, glassy eyes, eye deviation, nystagmus, blinking
Speech/cry	Weak or strong cry, grunting, hoarse, tone and inflection, speech pattern

T. B. Swan (✉)
Division of Pediatric Emergency Medicine, University of Florida, Gainesville, FL, USA
e-mail: tfalgiani@ufl.edu

A. Patel
Division of Emergency Medicine, Nemours Children's Hospital, University of Central Florida College of Medicine, Orlando, FL, USA
e-mail: amit.patel@nemours.org

C. M. Zeretzke-Bien, T. B. Swan (eds.), *Quick Hits for Pediatric Emergency Medicine*, https://doi.org/10.1007/978-3-031-32650-9_13

Signs of Altered Mental Status

- Poor responsiveness to environment or caregiver
- Weak or absent cry
- Eye deviation
- Abnormal pupillary size or reaction
- Abnormal respiratory patterns (tachypnea, apnea, Cheyne-Stokes respirations)
- Abnormal motor movements
- Lack of response to painful stimuli
- Irritability

Causes of Altered Mental Status in Children: AEIOU TIPS

A	Abuse
	Alcohol
	Arrythmia
	Acidosis
E	Electrolyte abnormality
	Encephalopathy
	Endocrine crisis
I	Infection
	Intussusception
	Intracranial hemorrhage
O	Overdose/ingestion
	Opiate ingestion
	Oxygen deprivation (hypoxia)
U	Uremia
T	Trauma
	Toxin
	Tumor
	Temperature (hyper or hypothermia)
I	Insulin-related issues (hyper/hypoglycemia, DKA)
	Inborn errors of metabolism
P	Psychosis
	Porphyria
	Psychogenic
S	Shock
	Seizures
	Stroke
	Shunt malfunction
	Syncope

General Treatment Guidelines

- ABCs: intubation for comatose or severely obtunded patients or inability to maintain/protect airway.
- Fluid bolus: 20 mL/kg if no cardiac etiology is suspected otherwise 10 mL/kg.
- Address and correct temperature abnormalities.
- Administer dextrose if hypoglycemic.
- Address and correct any electrolyte abnormalities.
- Consider naloxone.
- Avoid hypotension.
- Avoid hyperventilation.
- Obtain ECG.
- Administer broad spectrum antibiotics.
- Start specific therapy based on most likely diagnosis.

Initial Laboratory and Imagining Evaluation

- Bedside glucose, VBG or ABG, bedside electrolytes, CBC, blood culture, UA and urine culture, CSF studies and culture (if clinically stable), ammonia, complete metabolic panel, lactate, CRP, ESR.
- If inborn error of metabolism is suspected: obtain serum amino acids, urine organic acids, carnitine level.
- CT head if trauma suspected or visible, status epilepticus or severely obtunded.
- Consider toxicology screen.

Pediatric Altered Mental Status Pearls

1. Children may have subtle changes in their mental status. Utilize their caregivers and take their concerns seriously.
2. Always look for treatable causes, especially hypoglycemia.
3. Consider lead poisoning and Reye Syndrome in addition to infectious cause as an etiology of encephalopathy.
4. Consider EEG in the emergency department if patient remains in persistently altered state as some seizures may be undetectable by physical exam alone.
5. Toxic ingestion is still possible even if the toxicology screen is negative (many toxins do not show up on toxicology screen).
6. Non-accidental trauma should always be suspected as an etiology in all children with altered mental status.

Chapter 14
Pediatric Fever Protocols

Sakina Sojar, Colleen Gutman, Joon Choi, and Tricia B. Swan

Abstract Descriptive algorithms for the evaluation and management of the febrile neonate, infant, and child. The bacterial infection and ambulatory discharge disposition checklists are true "Quick Hits." Further risk stratification in the febrile child for a serious bacterial infection will improve resource utilization and breed antibiotic stewardship.

Well-appearing Febrile Infant: 0 to 21 days old

Exclusion Criteria: Ill Appearance, premature (< 37 weeks), chronic medical condition, focal infectious source (includes bronchiolitis, not URI)

Obtain the following labs:

Blood	Urine	CSF	Consider
Culture	Urinalysis	Gram stain	RVP
CBC, CMP	Culture	Cell count	HSV Testing (if
CRP,Procal	*specimen should be obtained by catheterization	Protein, glucose Meningitis PCR	risk factors)

Initiate Antibiotic Therapy
Ampicillin 100mg/kg q6h
Gentamicin 4mg/kg q24h*
*Should use ceftazidime (50 mg/kg q8h) if concern for meningitis
Add acyclovir if concern for HSV

Admit to Hospital

S. Sojar
Division of Pediatric Emergency Medicine, Department of Emergency Medicine, Warren Alpert Medical School of Brown University, Providence, RI, USA
e-mail: Sakina.sojar@brownphysicians.org

C. Gutman · J. Choi (✉) · T. B. Swan
Division of Pediatric Emergency Medicine, Department of Emergency Medicine, UF Health Shands Children's Hospital, University of Florida College of Medicine, Gainesville, FL, USA
e-mail: Ckays21@ufl.edu; Joonchoi@ufl.edu; tfalgiani@ufl.edu

Well-appearing Febrile Infant: 22 to 28 days old

Exclusion Criteria: Ill Appearance, premature (< 37 weeks), chronic medical condition, focal infectious source (includes bronchiolitis, not URI)

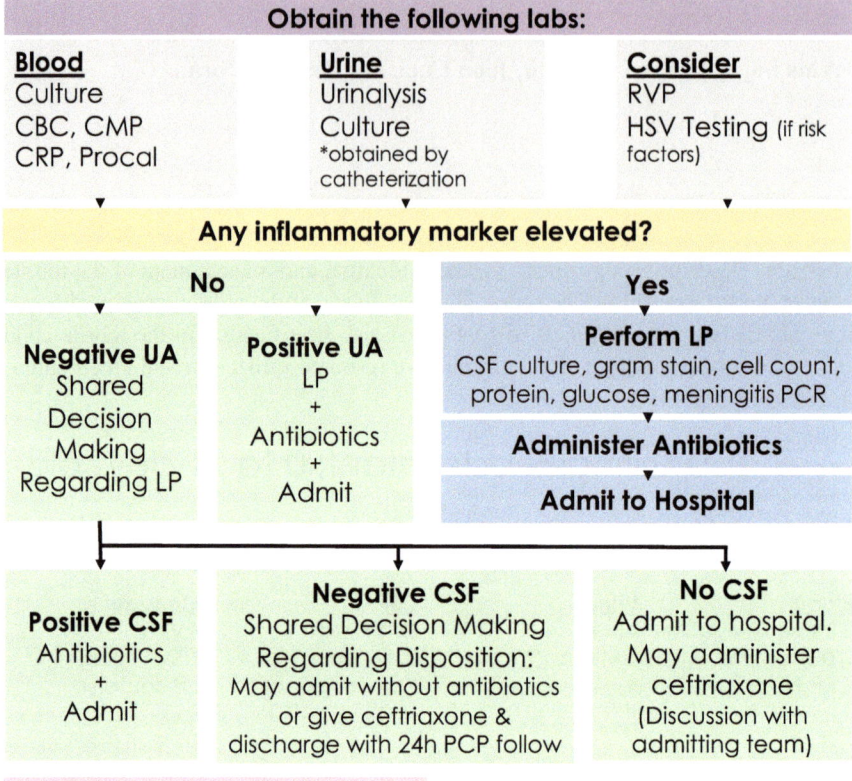

Obtain the following labs:

Blood
Culture
CBC, CMP
CRP, Procal

Urine
Urinalysis
Culture
*obtained by
catheterization

Consider
RVP
HSV Testing (if risk factors)

Any inflammatory marker elevated?

No

Yes

Negative UA
Shared Decision Making Regarding LP

Positive UA
LP
+
Antibiotics
+
Admit

Perform LP
CSF culture, gram stain, cell count, protein, glucose, meningitis PCR

Administer Antibiotics

Admit to Hospital

Positive CSF
Antibiotics
+
Admit

Negative CSF
Shared Decision Making Regarding Disposition:
May admit without antibiotics or give ceftriaxone & discharge with 24h PCP follow

No CSF
Admit to hospital. May administer ceftriaxone (Discussion with admitting team)

Definitions
Elevated Inflammatory Marker
- Temp > 38.5C
- CRP > 20 mg/L
- Procal > 0.5 ng/L
- ANC > 4000 per mm^3

Positive UA
- Any nitrite or LE
- WBC > 5 hpf

Positive CSF
- WBC > 8

Empiric Antibiotics
No defined source or UTI
Ceftriaxone 50mg/kg q24h
Meningitis
Ampicillin 100mg/kg
Ceftazidime 50mg/kg

Well-appearing Febrile Infant: 29 to 60 days old

Exclusion Criteria: Ill Appearance, premature (< 37 weeks), chronic medical condition, focal infectious source (includes bronchiolitis, not URI)

Obtain the following labs:

Blood	**Urine**	**Consider**
Culture	Urinalysis	RVP
CBC, CMP	Culture	HSV Testing (if risk factors)
CRP, Procal	*obtained by catheterization	

▼   ▼   ▼

Any inflammatory marker elevated?

No		**Yes**
▼	▼	▼

Positive UA	**Negative UA**	**Shared Decision Making Regarding LP**
Give ceftriaxone. Discharge with PO antibiotics and 24h PCP follow up	No antibiotics Discharge home w PCP follow up in 24 h	

Positive CSF	**Negative CSF**	**No CSF**
Antibiotics + Admit	UA Positive: Give ceftriaxone. May admit or discharge with PO antibiotics & 24h PCP follow up. UA Negative: May admit off antibiotics or discharge after ceftriaxone with 24h PCP follow up.	UA Positive: Administer ceftriaxone & admit to hospital. UA Negative: Admit to hospital. May administer ceftriaxone (Discussion with admitting team)

Definitions
Elevated Inflammatory Marker
- Temp > 38.5C
- CRP > 20 mg/L
- Procal > 0.5 ng/L
- ANC > 4000 per mm^3

Positive UA
- Any nitrite or LE
- WBC > 5 hpf

Positive CSF
- WBC > 8

Empiric Antibiotics
No defined source
Ceftriaxone 50mg/kg q24h
UTI only
Ceftriaxone 50mg/kg followed by:
Cefdinir 14mg/kg/day for 10 days
Meningitis
Ceftriaxone 100mg/kg q24h

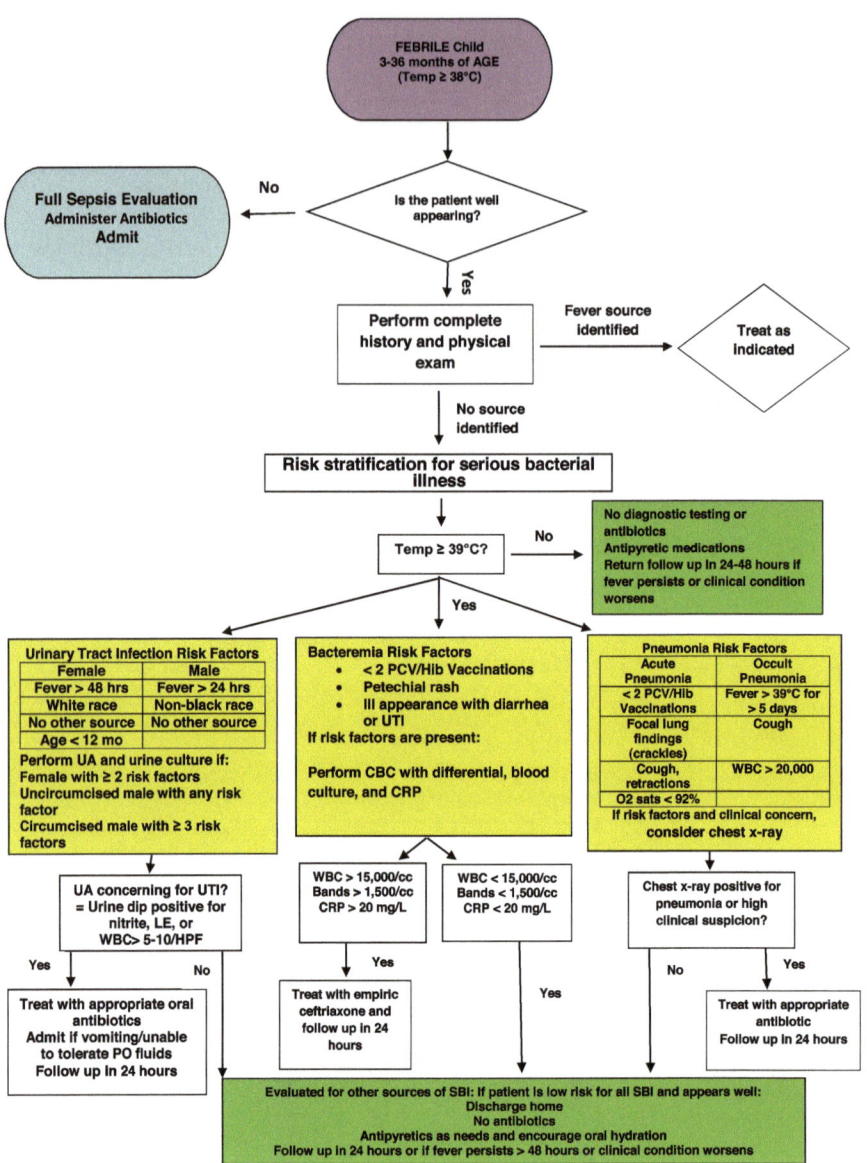

Quick Hits Pediatric Fever Pearls

1. Remember these algorithms only apply to the WELL-APPEARING infant!
2. Obtain inflammatory markers to facilitate decision-making.
3. Possible no lumbar puncture is necessary if 22–28 days old if inflammatory markers are negative.
4. In the 29–60 day old age range, shared decision making should be done regarding lumbar puncture if inflammatory markers are positive.
5. May discharge home if 22–28 days old if CSF is negative and ceftriaxone is given.
6. No antibiotics if 29–60 days old and urinalysis and inflammatory markers are negative.
7. All discharges should have close PCP follow-up (consider admission if cannot ensure).

Chapter 15
Pediatric Electrocardiography

Tricia B. Swan and Yiraima Medina-Blasini

Abstract This is what providers need to set them up for success interpreting a pediatric ECG, starting with special consideration and finishing with some pearls based on variation in age. The tables are full of Quick Hits based on ECG morphology and potential diagnosis that are crucial to the management of arrhythmias.

Special Considerations in Pediatric ECGs

- ECG normal values vary with age reflecting the changing anatomy of the growing heart.
- At birth the right ventricle is larger and thicker than the left ventricle which results in right axis deviation, T wave inversion in V1–V3, and prominent R wave in V1.
- Normal heart rate values are dependent on age.
- Conduction intervals are shorter (QRS duration, PR interval).
- To interpret pediatric ECGs accurately, it is important to have normal age-related value tables readily available.
- T wave inversion in V1–V3 may be a normal finding (juvenile T wave pattern).

T. B. Swan (✉)
Division of Pediatric Emergency Medicine, University of Florida, Gainesville, FL, USA
e-mail: tfalgiani@ufl.edu

Y. Medina-Blasini
Division of Pediatric Emergency Medicine, Department of Emergency Medicine, HCA Florida Kendall Hospital, Miami, FL, USA

Stepwise Approach to Interpretation of ECG: Rate, Rhythm, Axis, Intervals, and Voltages

Typical paper speed is 25 mm/s.

$$1\,mm = 1\,small\,box = 0.04\,s$$

$$5\,mm = 1\,large\,box = 0.2\,s$$

Rate

To calculate rate: 300 ÷ number of large squares between consecutive R waves.

Quick calculation: HR 300 = 1 large box, 150 = 2 large boxes, 100 = 3 large boxes, 75 = 4 large boxes, 60 = 5 large boxes.

Normal Heart Rate by Age

Age	Heart rate (bpm)
Premature	120–170
0–3 months	110–160
3–6 months	100–150
6–12 months	90–130
1–3 years	80–125
4–6 years	70–115
6 years to adult	60–100

Rhythm

- Sinus rhythm criteria:

    - Normal P wave (upright in I and aVF, inverted in aVR)
    - P wave before every QRS complex
    - QRS after every P wave
    - Constant PR interval

- Inversion of P wave in II or aVF indicates a low atrial rhythm (not sinus) or limb lead reversal.
- Sinus arrhythmia is a normal variant that causes rhythm variability with inspiration or expiration.

Axis (Fig. 15.1)

- The right ventricle is the dominant ventricle in the newborn and shifts the axis to the right (>90°).
- At 3–5 years of age the left ventricle catches up and then is the dominant ventricle and shifts the axis to the left (<90°).
- An abnormal axis can be one of the first clues for the diagnosis of congenital heart disease.
- Determine both P wave and QRS axes. Net summation of positive and negative deflections is used. Look for two perpendicular leads (usually lead I and AVF).

  – If QRS is positive in both lead I and AVF, the axis is in the left lower quadrant (0 − +90°).
  – If QRS is negative in lead I and positive in AVF, the axis is in the right lower quadrant (90–180°).

Fig. 15.1 Pediatric ECG axis

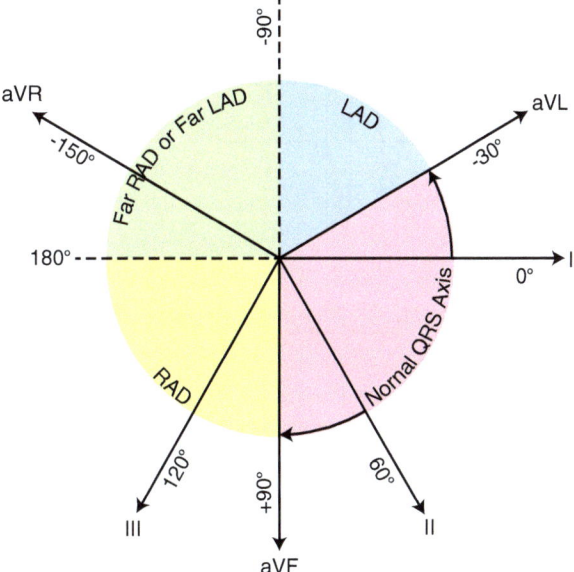

Normal QRS Axis by Age

Age	QRS axis
Birth to 1 month	+30 to 180°
1 month–3 years	+10 to 125°
4–5 years	0 to +110°
6–17 years	−15 to +110°
Adult	−30 to +105°

Adapted from Sharieff GQ, Rao SO. The Pediatric ECG. Emerg Med Clin North Am. 20,016; 24: 195–208

Intervals (Fig. 15.2)

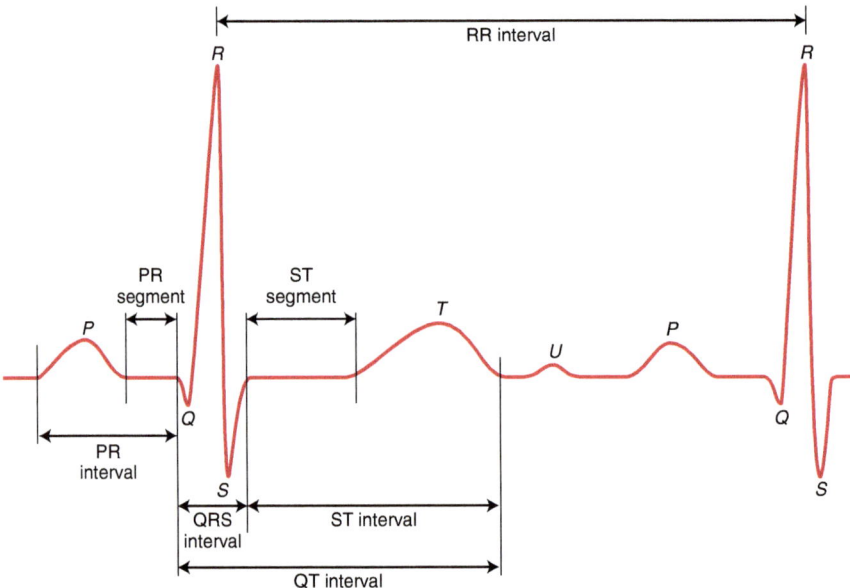

Fig. 15.2 Pediatric ECG intervals

PR Interval

- Measured from the beginning of the P wave to the beginning of the first deflection of the QRS complex.
- The PR interval is much shorter in neonates than in adults.

Normal PR Interval by Age

Age	PR interval (seconds)
Birth to 5 months	0.08–0.15
6 months–1 year	0.8–0.16
1–2 years	0.08–0.16
3–11 years	0.09–0.17
12–16 years	0.09–0.18
>16 years	0.12–0.20

Adapted from Sharieff GQ, Rao SO. The Pediatric ECG. Emerg Med Clin North Am. 20,016; 24: 195–208

Causes of Abnormalities of PR Interval

Prolonged PR interval	Shortened PR interval	Variable PR interval
Hyperkalemia	Pre-excitation pattern (WPW)	Wenckebach (Mobitz type 1)
Myocarditis	Glycogen storage disease	
Digitalis toxicity		
Certain congenital heart diseases (ASD, Ebstein)		
First degree AV block		

QRS Interval

- QRS interval lengthens as age increases.
- Abnormalities in the QRS morphology can detect ventricular hypertrophy which may reflect congenital heart disease.
- Right and left bundle branch patterns look similar to adult manifestations; however, the normal duration of the QRS interval is age related.
- In the presence of bundle branch block, determination of ventricular hypertrophy is difficult and an echocardiogram is indicated.
- Causes of prolonged QRS include bundle branch blocks, intraventricular block, ventricular arrhythmias, and pre-excitation syndromes (Wolff-Parkinson-White syndrome).

Normal QRS Interval by Age

Age	QRS interval (seconds)
Birth to 3 years	0.03–0.07
3–7 years	0.04–0.08
8–15 years	0.04–0.09
>16 years	0.05–0.10

Adapted from Sharieff GQ, Rao SO. The Pediatric ECG. Emerg Med Clin North Am. 20,016; 24: 195–208

QT Interval

- Diagnosis of prolonged QT is critical especially in the setting of seizures, syncope, or ALTE/BRUE events.
- Use the Bazett formula to correct the QT interval for heart rate:

  - Measured QT interval ÷ square root of the R-R interval.

Normal QTc Interval by Age

Age	QTc interval (seconds)
Birth to 1 week	0.47
1 week–6 months	0.45
> 6 months	0.44

Causes of Abnormalities of QTc

Prolonged QTc	Shortened QTc
Myocarditis	Congenital short QT syndrome
Ingestions/drugs (tricyclic antidepressants, ondansetron, antipsychotics)	Digitalis effect
Hypocalcemia	Hypercalcemia
Hypomagnesemia	
Head injury	
Long QT syndromes (Romano-Ward)	

Voltages (and Wave Morphology)

P Waves

- Should be upright in II and aVF and inverted in aVR.
- Normal P waves <3 mm tall

  - Tall P wave = right atrial enlargement

- Normal P wave duration

    - <0.07 s in infants
    - <0.09 s in children
    - Wide P wave = left atrial enlargement

- Tall and wide P wave = combined atrial hypertrophy

QRS Waves

Low QRS amplitude	High QRS amplitude
Pericarditis	Ventricular hypertrophy
Myocarditis	Ventricular conduction disturbances (WPW, bundle branch blocks)
Hypothyroidism	
Normal newborns	

- Age related-normal value tables are available for Q, R, and S waves.
- Recognition of ventricular hypertrophy:

    - Ventricular hypertrophy may be reflected by abnormalities in the QRS axis, QRS voltages, the R/S ratio, or T axis.
    - Evaluate QRS complex in V_1 and V_6. V_1 overlies the right ventricle and V_6 overlies the left ventricle, a tall R wave in these leads may mean hypertrophy.

Findings suggestive of RVH	Findings suggestive of LVH
Tall R wave in V_1 or V_2	Tall R wave in V_5 or V_6
Tall R wave in III and aVR	Tall R wave in I, II, aVL, aVR
Deep S wave in V_5/V_6	Deep S wave in V_1/V_2 or V4R
R/S ratio > upper limit of normal in V_1	R/S ratio > upper limit of normal in V_6
R/S ratio < lower limit of normal in V_6	R/S ratio < lower limit of normal in V_1
qR pattern in V1 (small Q wave, tall R wave)	Deep Q (>4 mm) in V_5/V_6
Upright T wave in V1 or V4R in children >3 days to 6 years (when T waves are normal otherwise)	Inverted T wave in V_6, I, and aVL
Right axis deviation for age	Left axis deviation for age

Q Waves

- Normal Q wave

    - Narrow (<0.04 s)
    - Less than 5 mm deep in aVF and left precordial leads
    - May be up to 8 mm deep in III in child <3 years old.

- Abnormal Q wave

    - Present in right precordial leads (i.e. V_1).
    - Absent in the left precordial leads.
    - Abnormally deep and/or wide (ventricular hypertrophy, MI, fibrosis)

ST Segment

- The normal ST-segment is isoelectric.
- ST-segment and T wave abnormalities signal similar pathology as in the adult ECG.
- J point (junction between QRS and ST segment) elevation and ST segment depression (2 mm in precordial leads/1 mm in limb leads) may be normal.
- Early repolarization (elevated ST segment and concave in leads with upright T wave) in adolescents is a normal variant.
- Ischemia, pericarditis, myocarditis, electrolyte disturbances, severe ventricular hypertrophy and digitalis effect may produce abnormalities.
- Pathologic ST changes:

    - Downward slope of ST segment followed by a biphasic inverted T wave.
    - Sustained horizontal ST segment depression ≥ 0.08 s.

T Waves

- T wave morphology changes with age

    - Birth to 1 week old, T waves are upright in the precordial leads.
    - After 1 week old, T waves typically inverted in V1–V3 (juvenile T wave pattern).
    - After 8 years old T waves become upright in V1–V3; however, juvenile T wave pattern may persist into early adulthood and can be a normal variant.

Causes of Abnormalities of T waves

Peaked T waves	Flat T waves	Inverted T waves
Hyperkalemia	Hypokalemia	Increased intracranial pressure
Early repolarization	Hypothyroidism	
LVH with volume overload	Pericarditis/myocarditis	
	Myocardial ischemia	
	Normal newborns	

Common ECG Findings Associated with Specific Diseases

Disease	ECG findings
Hypocalcemia	ST segment prolongation, prolonged QTc
Hypercalcemia	Shorted ST segment, shortened QTc
Hypokalemia	Prominent U waves, ST depression, biphasic or flat T waves, PR interval prolongation, SA block
Hyperkalemia	Peaked T waves, prolonged QRS, prolonged PR interval, absence of p waves, sine waves (wide, bizarre, biphasic QRS complex)
Myocardial infarction/ ischemia	ST elevation in contiguous leads with reciprocal ST depression, horizontal ST depression (ischemia)
Myocarditis	Low QRS voltage ($\leq$ 5 mm in limb leads), decreased T wave amplitude, QT prolongation, AV conduction disturbance (from PR prolongation to complete AV dissociation), deep Q waves and poor R wave progression in precordial leads, tachyarrhythmias
Pericarditis	QRS voltage <5 mm in limb leads, time dependent changes: PR segment depression and concave ST segment elevation→ST segment normalizes and flattened T waves→T wave inversion

Arrhythmias

Arrhythmia	ECG findings and characteristics	Management
Sinus tachycardia	• Rapid, regular sinus rhythm • Infants: < 220 bpm • Children: < 180 bpm • Common causes: Fever, sepsis, anemia, pain, hypovolemia, drug induced, pulmonary embolism	• Treat underlying cause
Supraventricular tachycardia (SVT)	• Rapid, regular, narrow (<80 ms) complex tachycardia (220–320 bpm in infants; 180–250 bpm in older children • P wave typically invisible; if visible will be abnormal in axis • P wave may be retrograde (follow QRS complex) • 90% of pediatric dysrhythmias are SVT and 90% of SVT are re-entrant type • ½ of children with SVT have no underlying heart disease (idiopathic) • ¼ of children will have congenital heart disease • ¼ of children will have WPW • Consider drug exposure or fever as cause • 2 types of SVT: Re-entrant and automatic • Do not use verapamil or beta-blockers in infants or children with SVT; may cause profound AV block, negative inotropy or sudden death	Vagal maneuvers: • Infants: Place ice on patient's face • Older children: valsalva maneuvers, carotid sinus massage Stable SVT • Adenosine (IV/IO) 0.1 mg/kg (first dose; max 6 mg), 0.2 mg/kg (second dose; max 12 mg). Unstable SVT (altered mental status, hypotension, or signs of shock) • Cardioversion 0.5–1 J/kg (max 2 J/kg) (consider sedation if cardioversion is going to be used)

Arrhythmia	ECG findings and characteristics	Management
Re-entrant SVT	• 90% of SVT • HR does not vary substantially • Begins and ends suddenly • Requires a bypass pathway (anatomic or functional) between atria and ventricles in addition to the AV node (e.g. WPW syndrome, AV nodal re-entrant tachycardia)	Antidromic • Drug of choice: Procainamide Orthodromic • Vagal maneuvers • Medications (IV/IO): Adenosine (first line) Procainamide[a] • Beta-blockers (metoprolol, propranolol, esmolol)[a]

Automatic SVT	• Abnormal or accelerated normal automaticity
	• Can be due to medications/drugs (e.g. sympathomimetics)
	• Begins and ends gradually
	• Includes
	  – Sinus tachycardia
	  – Atrial tachycardia
	  – Junctional ectopic tachycardia (usually post-atrial surgery)	

Wolf-Parkinson-White syndrome	• Occurrence of SVT plus
	  – Short PR interval
	  – Widened QS with slurred upstroke (delta wave)
	• Can cause wide complex tachycardia which may be mistaken for v tach (but is actually SVT with aberrancy)
		Long term treatment
		• Ablation
		• Cardiology consult

Ventricular tachycardia (V tach)	• Regular, fast heart rate • Widened QRS • Can be monomorphic or polymorphic • May be caused by prolonged QT • Extremely rare in children • Usually have history of congenital heart disease	Vtach with pulse • Adenosine IV/IO • Amiodarone IV/IO 5 mg/kg over 20 min • Procainamide IV/IO • 15 mg/kg over 30 min Pulseless • CPR/PALS algorithm • Defibrillation (2–4 J/kg) Followed by 2 min of high-quality CPR
Torsades de pointes	• Polymorphic ventricular tachycardia • Variable QRS amplitude • Associated with long QT syndrome (congenital or acquired, e.g. drug induced) • Patient can present with syncope or as a cardiac arrest • Can progress to ventricular fibrillation • Associated with sudden cardiac death in patients with long QT syndrome • Episode can be self-limited	With pulse • Magnesium sulfate 25–50 mg/kg IV bolus (max 2 gm/dose) • Unstable: synchronized cardioversion • Correct hypomagnesemia, hypokalemia, and/or hypocalcemia Pulseless • CPR/PALS algorithm • Defibrillation (2–4 J/kg) Followed by 2 min of CPR • Magnesium sulfate 25–50 mg/kg IV bolus (max 2 gm/dose)

Arrhythmia	ECG findings and characteristics	Management
Ventricular fibrillation (V fib)	• Chaotic irregular deflections of varying amplitude • No identifiable P waves, QRS complexes, or T waves • Rate 150–500 per minute • Amplitude decreases with duration (coarse VF - > fine VF) • Extremely rare in children • Usually have a history of congenital heart disease • Can be caused by prolonged QT, intracranial hemorrhage, medications	• CPR/PALS algorithm • Defibrillation 2–4 J/kg

IV intravenous, *IO* intraosseous
aShould be administered in consultation with pediatric cardiology specialist

Quick Hits Pediatric ECG Pearls

1. Interpretation of the pediatric ECG is challenging due to large variations in age-related normal values.
2. Use a stepwise approach to evaluate pediatric ECGs: rate, rhythm, axis, intervals, and voltages (or wave morphology).
3. Use reference tables to determine normal values for each age.
4. SVT is the most common arrhythmia in children.
5. Ninety-five percentage of wide complex tachycardias in children are NOT V tach but SVT with aberrancy or SVT with bundle branch block or accessory pathway re-entrant SVT.

Chapter 16
Pediatric Seizures

Tricia B. Swan and Todd Wylie

Abstract This chapter brings you a step-by-step guide on how to approach the actively seizing patient in status epilepticus. The differentiation of the simple versus complex febrile seizure is a must-know for all providers caring for the seizing pediatric patient. The differential diagnosis table of non-febrile seizures is a "Quick Hit" that can easily be accessed while difficult to remember.

T. B. Swan (✉)
Division of Pediatric Emergency Medicine, University of Florida, Gainesville, FL, USA
e-mail: Tfalgiani@ufl.edu

T. Wylie
Division of Pediatric Emergency Medicine, Department of Emergency Medicine, University of Florida College of Medicine-Jacksonville, Jacksonville, FL, USA
e-mail: Todd.wylie@jax.ufl.edu

Acute Management of Status Epilepticus

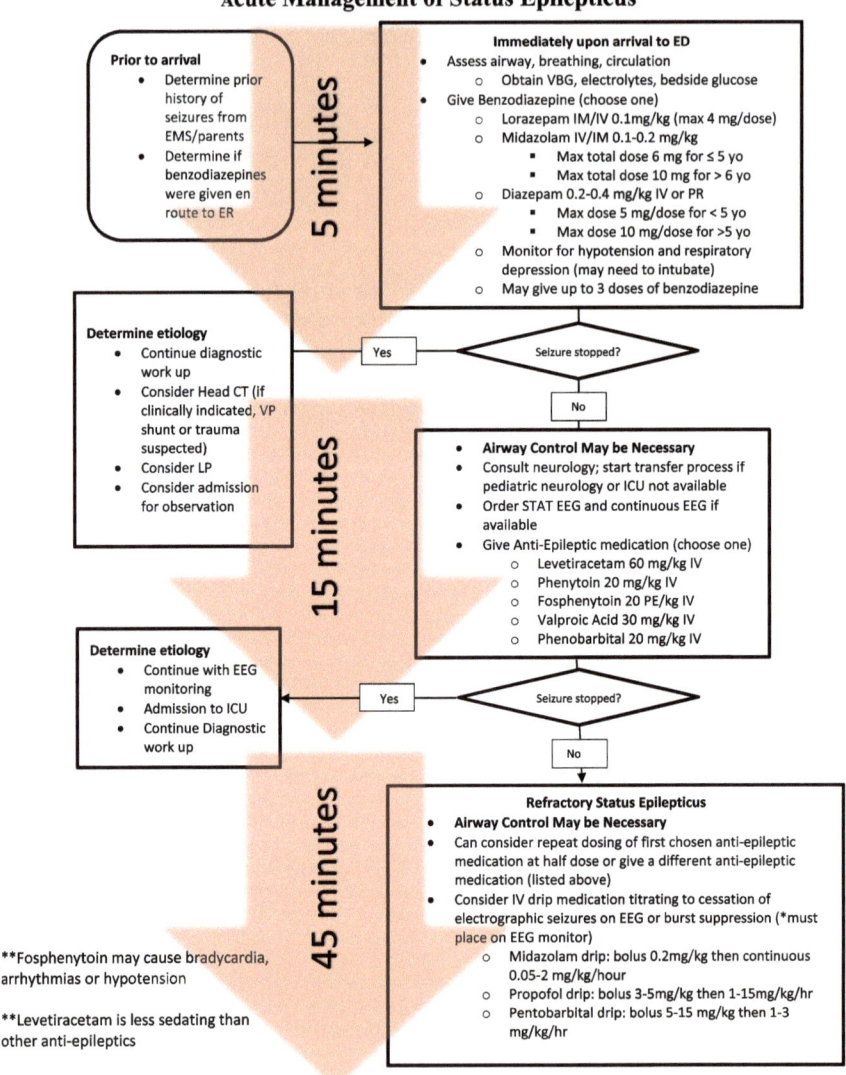

Acute Management of Status Epilepticus

Prior to arrival
- Determine prior history of seizures from EMS/parents
- Determine if benzodiazepines were given en route to ER

5 minutes

Immediately upon arrival to ED
- Assess airway, breathing, circulation
  - Obtain VBG, electrolytes, bedside glucose
- Give Benzodiazepine (choose one)
  - Lorazepam IM/IV 0.1mg/kg (max 4 mg/dose)
  - Midazolam IV/IM 0.1-0.2 mg/kg
    - Max total dose 6 mg for ≤ 5 yo
    - Max total dose 10 mg for > 6 yo
  - Diazepam 0.2-0.4 mg/kg IV or PR
    - Max dose 5 mg/dose for < 5 yo
    - Max dose 10 mg/dose for >5 yo
  - Monitor for hypotension and respiratory depression (may need to intubate)
  - May give up to 3 doses of benzodiazepine

Determine etiology
- Continue diagnostic work up
- Consider Head CT (if clinically indicated, VP shunt or trauma suspected)
- Consider LP
- Consider admission for observation

Yes ← Seizure stopped? → No

15 minutes

- **Airway Control May be Necessary**
- Consult neurology; start transfer process if pediatric neurology or ICU not available
- Order STAT EEG and continuous EEG if available
- Give Anti-Epileptic medication (choose one)
  - Levetiracetam 60 mg/kg IV
  - Phenytoin 20 mg/kg IV
  - Fosphenytoin 20 PE/kg IV
  - Valproic Acid 30 mg/kg IV
  - Phenobarbital 20 mg/kg IV

Determine etiology
- Continue with EEG monitoring
- Admission to ICU
- Continue Diagnostic work up

Yes ← Seizure stopped? → No

45 minutes

Refractory Status Epilepticus
- **Airway Control May be Necessary**
- Can consider repeat dosing of first chosen anti-epileptic medication at half dose or give a different anti-epileptic medication (listed above)
- Consider IV drip medication titrating to cessation of electrographic seizures on EEG or burst suppression (*must place on EEG monitor)
  - Midazolam drip: bolus 0.2mg/kg then continuous 0.05-2 mg/kg/hour
  - Propofol drip: bolus 3-5mg/kg then 1-15mg/kg/hr
  - Pentobarbital drip: bolus 5-15 mg/kg then 1-3 mg/kg/hr

**Fosphenytoin may cause bradycardia, arrhythmias or hypotension

**Levetiracetam is less sedating than other anti-epileptics

Defining Status Epilepticus

- Seizure lasting >5 min or repetitive seizure activity without return to neurologic baseline between seizures

- Early/impending status: 5 min
- Early stage status: 5–30 min
- Late/established status: 30–60 min
- Refractory status: Failure to respond to 2 doses of different antiepileptic drugs or duration >60 min

Treatment Goals for Status Epilepticus

1. Abort seizure (see algorithm above)

    (a) Antiepileptic drugs (AEDs) divided into agents for *emergent initial therapy, urgent control therapy,* and *refractory therapy.*

    - Emergent initial therapy: Benzodiazepines (lorazepam, midazolam, and diazepam) are primary agents and can be given IV, IM, IN, or PR depending on the agent.
    - Levetiracetam, fosphenytoin, phenobarbital, or valproic acid may also be considered for emergent initial therapy if seizure does not abort with benzodiazepines (after 3 doses).
    - Urgent control therapy: Levetiracetam, fosphenytoin, phenobarbital, or valproic acid.
    - Refractory therapy: Midazolam infusion, pentobarbital infusion, propofol infusion.

2. Airway management: Early airway control if seizure not rapidly aborted.
3. Maintain homeostasis and prevent cardiovascular collapse and brain injury.
4. Identify and treat underlying disorders.

Consideration of Underlying Disorders in Status Epilepticus

- Identify and correct any underlying electrolyte disturbance:
    - Hypoglycemia: give glucose.
    - Hyponatremia: give 3% NaCl.
    - Hypomagnesemia: give magnesium sulfate.
    - Hypocalcemia: give calcium gluconate.
- Consider pyridoxine deficiency (especially in neonatal seizure) or INH toxicity.
    - Give pyridoxine.
- Consider other toxidromes.
- Consider pregnancy.
- Consider hypoxia.

- Consider infectious etiology.
    - Broad spectrum antibiotics.
    - Acyclovir.
- Administer anti-pyretic if febrile.

Febrile Seizure Fundamentals

Simple	Complex
• T ≥ 38°C (100.4°F) • Age 6 mos-5 years • < 15 minute duration • Generalized • No recurrence in 24 hour time period	• T ≥ 38°C (100.4°F) • Age < 6 mo or > 5 years • > 15 minute duration • Focal features • Multiple seizures in 24 hours • 20-30% of all febrile seizures

Simple Febrile Seizures

- Definition: Seizure occurring between 6 months and 5 years of age that is associated with a fever (temp greater than 38 °C) but without evidence of CNS infection or other defined neurologic disease.
- Simple febrile seizures (85%) are more common than complex febrile seizures.
- There is a family history of febrile seizures in immediate family members in 25–40% of cases.
- Very low risk of meningitis.
- Not the SOLE indication of meningitis.
- No difference in risk of serious bacterial illness compared with febrile kids who do not seize.
- Neuroimaging not indicated for routine evaluation.

- EEG not typically indicated for routine evaluation.
- Labs only as indicated for evaluation of fever cause.
- LP should be considered if: signs or symptoms suggesting CNS infection are present, 6mo–12mo and unimmunized or immunization status is deficient or unclear, pre-treatment/receiving treatment with systemic antibiotics or does not return to neurologic baseline.
- **Management**

  – Acetaminophen has potential to prevent recurrent febrile seizures during same fever episode.
  – Long-term anticonvulsant medications are not recommended for children with a simple febrile seizure.

- **Consequences of simple febrile seizures**

  – Increased risk of recurrent febrile seizures (approximately 33% recurrence risk).
  – Slightly increased risk of subsequent afebrile seizures compared to general population.

Complex Febrile Seizures

- Even in complex febrile seizures rate of acute bacterial meningitis is LOW, though higher risk in comparison with simple febrile seizures.
- Rarely the SOLE indicator of meningitis.
- Diagnostic evaluation difficult due to heterogeneity of presentation.
- Neuroimaging indicated for any of the following:

  – Focal seizure
  – Prolonged seizure
  – Persistent altered mental status
  – Focal findings on examination
  – Signs or symptoms of increased intracranial pressure
  – Macrocephaly

- LP or No LP?

  – Threshold to perform LP should be lower.
  – LP for persistent altered mental status, focal neuro exam, or clinical concern.
  – LP for unimmunized or incomplete vaccination status.
  – LP if patient has been treated/partially pre-treated with antibiotics.
  – Strongly consider observation admission.

Evaluation of First Time Non-febrile Seizure

- Most require ONLY a complete history and physical! Do only H&P for HEALTHY children back to baseline (no labs or imagining!).
- Younger children, not back to baseline or underlying diseases may need more investigation.
- Utilize risk factors to guide when you should perform neuroimaging (CT or MRI):

  - Abnormal or focal neurologic exam
  - Predisposing history (sickle cell disease, bleeding disorder, cerebral vascular disease, cancer, HIV, hemihypertrophy, hydrocephalus, closed head injury, VP shunt or recent shunt revision, travel to areas with endemic cysticercosis)
  - Focal seizure or focal manifestations
  - Persistent altered mental status or status epilepticus
  - Age < 6 months
  - Uncertain follow-up
  - Suspicion for non-accidental trauma

- Get labs for

  - Kids under 6 months of age (including ionized calcium)
  - History of diabetes or other metabolic disorder
  - Suggestive clinical history (vomiting, diarrhea)
  - Persistent altered mental status
  - Status epilepticus

- Lumbar puncture

  - No evidence supporting routine performance of LP
  - NOT for the well child that has returned back to baseline neurologic status
  - Only if clinically indicated
  - LP should be done in ALL neonates (<28 days old).

- Should perform an EEG (can be done as outpatient at a follow neurology visit).
- Disposition:

  - Back to normal: discharge home (arrange outpatient EEG).
  - Education for families: what to do if seizure occurs.
  - Outpatient follow-up with pediatric neurologist.
  - Activity restrictions! (No swimming alone, no bathing alone, no driving, no mountain climbing, driving ATVs, etc.)
  - Does not need antiepileptic medication.

Differential diagnosis of non-febrile seizures
Breath holding
Syncope
Non-accidental trauma
Encephalopathy
Parasomnia
TICs
Hypoglycemia
Complex migraine
Arrhythmia
Benign myoclonus of infancy
Gastroesophageal reflux (Sandifer syndrome)
Chills
Psychogenic non-epileptic seizures (PNES)

Neonatal Seizures (≤ 28 Days of Age)

- Full septic workup (CBC, blood culture, UA, urine culture, CSF studies and CSF culture)
- HSV surface cultures
- CSF HSV
- Obtain electrolytes.
- Obtain imagining (CT or brain MRI).
- Give antibiotics and acyclovir (cover meningitis and HSV meningitis).
- Give pyridoxine (50–100 mg) if seizure is intractable.

Quick Hit Pediatric Seizure Management Pearls

1. Benzodiazepines are the initial drug of choice for the treatment of seizures and can be administered IV, IM, IN, or PR.
2. **Simple Febrile Seizure: Bottom Line**
   (a) Treat like any other kid with fever.
   (b) LP if concerned for meningitis or physical exam findings concerning for meningitis.
   (c) LP is an *OPTION* if un/under-immunized or pre-treatment with antibiotics.

3. **Complex Febrile Seizures: Bottom Line**

   (a) Lower threshold to tap.
   (b) Do NOT need to perform LP in the WELL appearing child who is back to baseline.
   (c) Strongly consider observation admission.

4. **First Non-Febrile Seizure: MUST DO:**

   (a) Clinical exam
   (b) History
   (c) Education/activity restrictions!
   (d) Everything else DEPENDS on clinical exam or concerning history findings.
   (e) Basic labs and imaging in <6 months of age or predisposing conditions.
   (b) Overall labs, LP, EEG, and imaging are NOT needed in the ED; will need outpatient EEG.

Chapter 17
Electrolyte Disturbances

Tricia B. Swan and Carmen J. Martinez

Abstract This electrolyte disturbances chapter is full of important pearls to the identification and treatment of hyponatremia, hypernatremia, hypokalemia, hyperkalemia, hypokalemia, and hypoglycemia. The tables are a vital tool to help identify the etiology of the patient's electrolyte abnormality. Treatments are concise and bulleted for quick reference and action.

Hyponatremia ($Na^+ < 135$ mEq/L)

Signs/Symptoms

- Altered mental status
- Lethargy
- Seizures
- Coma
- Decreased tendon reflexes
- Hypothermia
- Respiratory distress or respiratory failure, Cheyne-stokes respirations
- Anorexia
- Nausea, vomiting
- Muscle cramps
- Weakness
- Agitation
- Headaches

T. B. Swan (✉)
Division of Pediatric Emergency Medicine, University of Florida, Gainesville, FL, USA
e-mail: tfalgiani@ufl.edu

C. J. Martinez
Division of Pediatric Emergency Medicine, Department of Emergency Medicine, USA Health Children's and Women's Hospital, University of South Alabama, Mobile, AL, USA
e-mail: cmartinez@health.southalabama.edu

Type	Etiology	Notable laboratory findings	Treatment
Pseudohyponatremia	Hyperlipidemia (Na^+ decreased by $0.002 \times$ lipid mg/dL) Hyperproteinemia (Na^+ decreased by $0.25 \times$ [protein g/dL-8])	Normal serum osmolality	Treat underlying cause
Pseudohyponatremia	Hyperglycemia (Na^+ decreased by 1.6 mEq/L for each 100 mg/dL rise in glucose over 100) Mannitol infusion	High serum osmolality	Treat underlying cause
Renal loss	Diuretics Adrenal insufficiency Na^+-losing nephropathy Obstructive uropathy Renal tubular acidosis Cerebral salt wasting	Decreased weight ↑ Urine volume ↑ Urine Na^+ ↓ Urine osmolality ↓ Urine specific gravity	Treat underlying cause Replace losses
Extrarenal loss	GI losses (diarrhea, vomiting) Skin losses Cystic fibrosis Third spacing (ascites, burns, pancreatitis, etc.)	Decreased weight ↓ Urine volume ↓ Urine Na^+ ↑ Urine osmolality ↑ Urine specific gravity	Treat underlying cause Replace losses
Other	SIADH Congestive heart failure Nephrotic syndrome Acute or chronic renal failure Water intoxication Improper formula mixing Cirrhosis Hypothyroidism	Increased or normal weight ↓ Urine volume ↓ Urine Na^+ ↑ Urine osmolality ↑ Urine specific gravity	Treat underlying cause Restrict fluids/free water

Emergent Management for Hyponatremia

- Treat symptomatic hyponatremia (seizures, coma, etc.) with IV hypertonic saline:

  - Give 4–6 mL/kg of 3% NaCl.
  - Each mL/kg of 3% NaCl will increase the serum Na^+ by approximately 1 mEq/L.
  - Do not increase the serum Na^+ to more than 130 mEq/L acutely.

- Rapid correction of hyponatremia can cause central pontine myelinolysis:

  - Avoid increasing the serum Na^+ more than 12 mEq/L every 24 h.

- Treat asymptomatic hyponatremia with identification of underlying cause and then disease-specific treatment such as fluid and sodium replacement, water restriction, hormone replacement, or dialysis.

Hypernatremia (Na⁺ > 145 mEq/L)

Signs/Symptoms

- Altered mental status
- Lethargy
- Seizures
- Coma
- Decreased tendon reflexes
- Hyperthermia
- Respiratory distress or respiratory failure
- Nausea, vomiting
- Muscle cramps
- Weakness
- Irritability
- Headaches

Type	Etiology	Notable laboratory findings	Treatment
Renal loss	Diuretics Diabetes insipidus Nephropathy Post-obstructive diuresis Acute tubular necrosis (diuretic phase)	Decreased weight ↑ Urine volume ↑ Urine Na⁺ ↓ urine specific gravity	Treat underlying cause Replace free water loss
Extrarenal loss	GI losses (diarrhea, vomiting) Skin losses Respiratory loss of free water Insensible losses (premature infant, radiant warmers, phototherapy)	Decreased weight ↓ Urine volume ↓ Urine Na⁺ ↑ Urine specific gravity	Treat underlying cause Replace free water loss
Other	Mineralocorticoid excess Hyperaldosteronism Exogenous Na⁺ intake Improper formula mixing Administration of sodium containing medications or fluids (sodium bicarbonate, hypertonic saline) Seawater ingestion Inadequate oral intake (ineffective breastfeeding, child abuse/neglect, etc.)	Increased weight ↓ Urine volume ↓ Urine Na⁺ ↑ urine osmolality ↑ Urine specific gravity	Treat underlying cause Replace free water loss Stop exogenous intake or administration of sodium containing medications or fluids

Emergent Management for Hypernatremia

- Identify and treat underlying cause.
- Stop exogenous administration of any sodium containing fluids/medications.
- For patients with shock or severe dehydration, volume expansion with isotonic saline is recommended **regardless** of serum Na$^+$.
- Hypernatremia should not be corrected rapidly:
  Serum Na$^+$ should not be lowered more than 10–12 mEq/L per 24 h.

Hypokalemia (K < 3.5 mEq/L)

Signs/Symptoms

- Muscle weakness
- Muscle cramps
- Paralysis
- Ileus/constipation
- Areflexia
- Arrhythmias
- Respiratory distress
- Urinary retention

ECG changes: flattened or absent T wave, ST segment depression, presence of a U wave between T wave and P wave, ventricular fibrillation, Torsades de Pointes.

Etiologies	
Decreased intake	Anorexia nervosa
	Poor diet (rare)
Transcellular shift	Alkalosis
	Insulin therapy
	Albuterol therapy
	Familiar hypokalemic periodic paralysis
Renal loss	Renal tubular acidosis
	Diuretics
	DKA
	Excessive mineralocorticoid effect (Bartter's syndrome, Cushing syndrome, licorice ingestion, hyperaldosteronism)
	Acute tubular necrosis
	Fanconi syndrome
	Antibiotics (high urine anions, especially penicillins)

Etiologies	
Extrarenal loss	Vomiting/excessive NG suction
	Pyloric stenosis
	Cystic fibrosis
	Diarrhea
	Laxative abuse
	Ureterosigmoidostomy
	Excessive sweating
Spurious	Leukocytosis

Emergent Management for Hypokalemia

- Obtain ECG.
- Obtain creatine kinase (CK) (hypokalemia can cause rhabdomyolysis); glucose; ABG; urinalysis; urine K^+, Na^+, and Cl^-; and urine osmolality.
- If respiratory paralysis or cardiac arrhythmia is present, infuse 1 mEq/kg/h.
- If patient is not critical, calculate K^+ deficit, and replace with potassium acetate or potassium chloride. Oral replacement is safer when feasible.
- Correct underlying causes (DKA, alkalosis, etc.).
- If IV replacement is necessary, no more than 40 mEq/L via peripheral route or 80 mEq/L via central route should be used.

Hyperkalemia (K > 5.5 mEq/L)

Signs/Symptoms

- Muscle weakness
- Paresthesias
- Paralysis
- Areflexia
- Arrhythmias
- Respiratory distress

ECG changes: ECG changes progress with increasing serum K^+ levels. Peaked T waves, prolongation PR interval, loss of P waves with widening QRS, amplified R wave, progressive widening of QRS, bradycardia, AV block, ventricular arrhythmias, Torsades de Pointes, sinus wave pattern (wide QRS merging with T wave), cardiac arrest.

Etiologies	
Increased intake	IV or PO medications
	Exogenous K^+ intake (salt substitutes)
	Transfusions with aged blood
Transcellular shift	Acidosis
	Rhabdomyolysis
	Tumor lysis syndrome
	Large hematomas
	Succinylcholine
	Exercise
	Insulin deficiency
	Malignant hyperthermia
	Hyperkalemic periodic paralysis
	Crush injuries, trauma, burns
Decreased renal excretion	Renal failure
	Congenital adrenal hyperplasia
	K^+-sparing diuretics
	Renal tubular diseases
	Urinary tract obstruction
	Aldosterone insensitivity
	Aldosterone deficiency
	Lupus nephritis
	Medications
Spurious	Hemolysis
	Thrombocytosis
	Leukocytosis
	Tight tourniquet during lab draw

Emergent Management for Hyperkalemia

- Obtain ECG.
- Continuous cardiac monitoring.
- Obtain repeat specimen; do not delay treatment waiting on repeat lab results!
- Stop all K^+ infusions or medications.
- If ECG changes are present:

   - IV administration of 10–20 mg/kg (max 500 mg) calcium chloride or 100 mg/kg/dose (max dose 3 g/dose) calcium gluconate over 5 min to stabilize cardiac membrane.
   - **Patient must remain on cardiac monitor and infusion stopped if HR < 60, (bradycardia can be fatal).**
   - Shift K^+ intracellularly:

      Give IV sodium bicarbonate 1–2 mEq/kg over 5–10 min (if metabolic acidosis is present).
      Give 5 mg nebulized albuterol.
      Give IV insulin + glucose infusion (must give glucose with insulin therapy to prevent hypoglycemia).

- Initiate dialysis if renal failure.
- Kayexalate 1 g/kg PO or PR to bind K+ (does not work immediately).
- Give mineralocorticoids if deficiency is suspected.
- Correct any co-existing magnesium deficiency.

Hypocalcemia (Ca^{++} < 7 mg/dL in Preterm Infant, <8 mg/dL in Term Infant, or < 9 mg/dL in Children)

Signs/Symptoms

- Muscular irritability
- Weakness
- Tetany
- Paresthesias
- Fatigue
- Muscle cramps
- Altered mental status
- Seizures
- Laryngospasm
- Cardiac arrhythmias
- Prolonged QT interval
- Trousseau sign (carpopedal spasm after arterial occlusion)
- Chvostek sign (perioral twitch with stimulus of the facial nerve)

Etiologies

Early Neonatal (1-3 days)	Late Neonatal (3 days- 6 weeks)	Infants/Children
• Prematurity	• Hypoparathyroidism	• Hypoparathyroidsim
• Poor intake/delayed feeds	• Maternal hypercalcemia	• Autoimmune disease
• Increased calcitonin	• DiGeorge Syndrome	• Vitamin D deficiency (espicially if strictly breastfeeding without supplementation)
• Hypoxic encephalopathy	• Velo-cardio-facial Syndrome	• Wilson's disease
• Neonatal asphyxia	• Cow's milk tetany (high phosphate load with cow's milk)	• Hyperphospatemia from improper forumla mixing
• Intrauterin growth restriction	• Chronic diarrhea	• Excessive use of phosphorus containing enemas
• Exchange transfusion (citrate load)	• Malabsorption	• Total parental nutrition (TPN)
• Infant of a diabetic mother	• Alkaline treatements	• Blood transfusion
• Hypomagnesemia	• Hypomagnesemia	• Chelation therapy
• Hypoalbunemia	• Severe infantile osteopetrosis	• Acute severe illness
• Maternal hyperparathyroidism	• Renal disease	• Malabsorption
• Dietary phosphate loading		• Pancreatitis
		• Respiratory or metabolic alkalosis
		• Renal disease/renal failure
		• Hypomagnesemia
		• Medications

Emergent Management for Hypocalcemia

- Obtain ECG (causes arrhythmias/prolonged QT).
- Obtain total and ionized Ca^{++} levels, phosphate level, alkaline phosphatase, magnesium level, total protein, complete metabolic profile, 25-OH vitamin D, parathyroid hormone (PTH) level, albumin, ABG (acidosis increased ionized calcium), chest X-ray to visualize the thymus, ankle and wrist X-rays to assess for rickets, and urine studies for calcium, phosphate, and creatinine.
- Correct hypomagnesemia first if present (if $mg^{++} < 1.5$ mg/dL) before calcium infusion.
- Stop any medication or infusions that may bind calcium (blood transfusions, TPN).
- Treatment for severe tetany, seizures, or cardiac arrhythmias:

  - 10% IV calcium gluconate 100 mg/kg given slowly over 10 min.
  - **Patient must remain on cardiac monitor and infusion stopped if HR < 60 (bradycardia can be fatal).**
  - Never mix calcium with fluids containing phosphate or bicarbonate.

- If patient is stable, replacement therapy can be oral.
- Address and treat any underlying causes.

Hypercalcemia ($Ca^{++} > 11$ mg/dL)

Signs/Symptoms

- Muscular irritability
- Weakness
- Lethargy
- Altered mental status/coma
- Seizures
- Abdominal cramping
- Cardiac arrhythmias
- Shortened QT interval
- Polyuria
- Polydipsia
- Pancreatitis
- Renal calculi
- Nausea, vomiting, anorexia

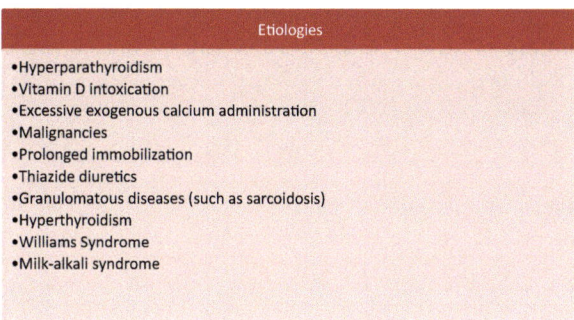

Etiologies
•Hyperparathyroidism •Vitamin D intoxication •Excessive exogenous calcium administration •Malignancies •Prolonged immobilization •Thiazide diuretics •Granulomatous diseases (such as sarcoidosis) •Hyperthyroidism •Williams Syndrome •Milk-alkali syndrome

Emergent Management for Hypercalcemia

- Obtain ECG (causes arrhythmias/shortened QT).
- Obtain total and ionized Ca^{++} levels; phosphate level; alkaline phosphatase; total protein; complete metabolic profile; 25-OH vitamin D; parathyroid hormone (PTH) level; albumin; urine studies for calcium, phosphate, and creatinine; abdominal X-ray; renal ultrasound to assess for renal calculi.
- Address and treat any underlying causes.
- Hydration to increase urine output and Ca^{++} elimination, may give NS boluses for rapid hydration.
- Furosemide for diuresis.
- Severe or refractory hypercalcemia may require dialysis.

Hypoglycemia (Glucose <50 mg/dL)

Signs/Symptoms

- Diaphoresis
- Tachycardia
- Pallor
- Trembling/jitteriness
- Headache
- Confusion
- Altered mental status
- Lethargy

- Apnea
- Nausea, vomiting
- Difficulty speaking
- Weakness
- Seizures
- Ataxia
- Vision changes
- Poor feeding

Etiologies	
Glucose use increased	Hyperinsulinism: Insulin-producing tumor, ingestion of oral hypoglycemic agent, insulin therapy or overdose Large tumors (e.g., Wilms', neuroblastoma) Hyperthermia Growth hormone deficiency Polycythemia Infant of diabetic mothers

Glucose availability decreased	Decreased oral intake
	Fasting
	Malnutrition
	Diarrhea
	Vomiting
	Inborn errors of metabolism
	    Inability to mobilize glucose
	    Ineffective gluconeogenesis
	    Inadequate glycogen reserve
	    Ineffective glycogenolysis

Availability of alternative fuel decreased	Low/absent fat stores Enzyme deficiency in fatty acid oxidation
Others	Sepsis Shock Cardiogenic shock Burns Reye's syndrome Medications Salicylate ingestion Alcohol ingestion Other ingestions (esp. cardiac meds) Adrenal insufficiency Hypothyroidism Panhypopituitarism Hepatitis/liver failure

Emergent Management for Hypoglycemia

- **Immediate treatment of hypoglycemia: Rule of 50 (dextrose fluid × mL/ kg = 50):**
  - **D50 = 1 mL/kg fluid bolus**
  - **D25 = 2 mL/kg fluid bolus**
  - **D10 = 5 mL/kg fluid bolus**
  - **D5 = 10 mL/kg fluid bolus**
- Once initial hypoglycemia has been corrected, begin infusion with D10-containing fluids at 1.5–2 × MIVF rate.
- Administer stress dose of glucocorticoid (2 mg/kg of hydrocortisone).
- Laboratory studies: CBC, blood culture, complete metabolic panel, ammonia, glucagon, c-peptide, lactate, pyruvate, carnitine level, ABG, acylcarnitine profile, cortisol level, growth hormone, plasma amino acids, urine organic acids, urinalysis, urine culture.
- Do not delay therapy with dextrose in order to obtain labs: Give glucose immediately!
- Inborn errors of metabolism/genetic disorders and ingestion should be high on your differential diagnosis in infants or children presenting with hypoglycemia.

Quick Hits Electrolyte Disturbances Pearls

1. Rapid correction of hyponatremia can cause central pontine myelinolysis, avoid increasing the serum Na^+ more than 12 mEq/L every 24 h.
2. For patients with shock or severe dehydration with hypernatremia, volume expansion with isotonic saline is recommended regardless of serum Na^+.
3. For patients receiving IV calcium infusions, they must remain on cardiac monitor and infusion stopped if HR <60 (bradycardia can be fatal)!
4. Prompt recognition and treatment of hypoglycemia in children is critical: remember the "rule of 50" for dextrose administration!

Chapter 18
Pediatric Toxicology

Judith K. Lucas

Abstract One pill can kill in a pediatric ingestion. You must know the antidote and be able to identify a corresponding toxidrome to stabilize and manage a potentially lethal condition. This chapter leads you through the most common ingestions and antidotes in an easy-to-read table format. The commonly used acronyms are a "Quick Hit" that most providers struggle to remember. The button battery ingestion algorithm is extremely high yield and an excellent reference for management versus emergent transfer.

Management of ALL Pediatric Poisonings Should Include Consultation with the Poison Control Center. Call 1–800–222-1222 (Nationwide)

Children <6 Years Old Make Up 48.6% of all Human Exposures

Top 10 *exposures* in children < 6 years of age	Top 10 *fatalities* in children < 6 years of age
Cosmetics	Fumes, gasses, vapors
Cleaning substances (household)	Analgesics (methadone, hydromorphone)
Analgesics	Household cleaners
Foreign bodies/toys/miscellaneous	Alcohols
Topical preparations	Antihistamines
Vitamins	Cardiovascular medications
Antihistamines	Cosmetics/personal care products
Pesticides	Sedative/hypnotics
Gastrointestinal preparations	Miscellaneous
Plants	Button batteries

J. K. Lucas (✉)
Division of Pediatric Emergency Medicine, Department of Emergency Medicine, UF Health Shands Children's Hospital, University of Florida College of Medicine, Gainesville, FL, USA
e-mail: judithklucas@ufl.edu

Toxidromes

Toxidrome	HR	RR	Sys BP	Temp	Mental status	Pupils	GI[a]	Skin
Sympathomimetic	↑	↑	↑	↑	Agitated	Dilated	↑	Diaphoretic
Anticholinergic	↑	↑	↑	↑	Agitated Seizures Impaired	Dilated	↓	Dry
Cholinergic	±	± (bronchorrhea)	±	−	Agitated Impaired	±	↑	Diaphoretic
Opioid	↓	↓	↓	↓	Impaired	Pinpoint	↓	−

[a]GI: Upward arrow indicates increased peristalsis, with associated increased bowel sounds; downward arrow indicates decreased peristalsis, to point of ileus, with associated decreased or absent bowel sounds

Small Doses, Big Problems

Several medications in small doses or single pill are toxic, or even lethal in children.

***Suspected ingestion of any of these substances should include observation up to 24 h even in asymptomatic pediatric population.

Drug	Toxicity	Management
Benzocaine/Prilocaine (over the counter)	Local anesthetic (teething gels, EMLA) Ingestion, mucosal, or dermal absorption Onset 30–60 min, up to 6 h Methemoglobinemia: Symptoms dependent on methemoglobin concentration • Cyanosis without signs of symptoms (levels <30%) • CV compromise as methemoglobin levels rise	**Antidote:** Methylene blue 1–2 mg/kg, with repeat dosing Q 1 h (max of 7 mg/kg)
Camphor (over the counter)	Found in topical ointments Symptom onset: 10–20 min post-ingestion Neurotoxic: excitatory, seizures with subsequent progression to coma and respiratory depression	A, B, C's Decontaminate the skin Seizures: give benzodiazepines/ barbiturates

Drug	Toxicity	Management
Calcium channel blockers	**Bradycardia, hypotension, hyperglycemia: think Calcium Channel blockers!** Worse with phenylalkylamines (verapamil) • Cardiovascular disturbance • Hypotension and bradycardia • Second and third degree block • Cardiogenic shock secondary to extreme negative inotropy • Decreased mental status seizures • Hyperglycemia	A, B, C's Volume Inotropes Ability to perform transcutaneous pacing *Consider* activated charcoal (1 gm/kg, up to 50 gm) if within 1 h and airway protected **Antidotes:** Glucagon, 50 µg/kg initial bolus, double subsequent doses if no effect (max dose is 10 mg) Calcium chloride, 10–25 mg/kg 10% CaCl IV q 10–20 min (max 1 gm) Glucose + insulin
Clonidine (and the imidazolines)	Includes VISINE^R (tetrahydrozoline) CLEAR EYES^R (naphazoline) (*over the counter*) Includes the CLONIDINE PATCH, as well as oral formulations Opioid toxidrome: • Bradycardia • Respiratory depression • Symptoms may be prolonged and recurrent for up to 24 h	A, B, C's Volume Atropine, 0.02 mg/kg, Q 20 min for symptomatic bradycardia **Antidote:** Narcan, 0.1 mg/kg IV/ ETT/SC/IN/IM/IO, given every 2 min. Up to a max or 2 mg *may* be helpful; higher doses than usual may be required
Cyclic antidepressants	All potent inhibitors of norepi uptake; many inhibit serotonin uptake as well Classic EKG finding: QRS interval prolongation • Tachydysrhythmias: V tach • Torsades de pointes Seizures Anticholinergic toxidrome	A, B, C'S Ability to perform transcutaneous pacing *Consider* activated charcoal (1 gm/kg, up to 50 g) if presents within first hour, there are bowel sounds, and the airway is secure Benzodiazepines/ barbiturates for seizures **Antidote**: Sodium bicarbonate Initial bolus: 1–2 mEq/kg for QRS > 100 ms Sodium bicarbonate infusion: goal to achieve a serum pH of 7.5

Drug	Toxicity	Management
Diphenoxylate hydrochloride/Atropine sulfate	(LOMOTIL[R]): unique opiate/ anticholinergic combination *No correlation between dose ingested and the severity of toxicity* Symptoms may present in first hour, OR be delayed by >12 h Toxicity may have components of both anticholinergic toxidrome and opioid toxidrome Symptoms may persist for up to 30 h, with *recurrence of respiratory and CNS depression*	A, B, Cs Volume Respiratory and ventilator support **Antidote:** Naloxone, 0.1 mg/kg IV/ ETT/SC/IN/IM/IO, given every 2 min. Up to a max or 2 mg *may* be helpful; higher doses than usual may be required
Methyl salicylate- (*over the counter*)	Severe, rapid-onset salicylate toxicity due to its high concentration; found in arthritis rubs and oil of wintergreen 1 mL oil of wintergreen = 1.4 gm aspirin (5 mL = 7 g!) As little as 4 mL in a child can be fatal Symptom onset rapid, usually within 2 h post-ingestion • GI: Nausea, vomiting, and abdominal pain; hematemesis • Tinnitus • Acid-base disturbances • Hypoglycemia • Hyperthermia • seizures, coma	Immediate ASA level (unlike with acetaminophen) Serial charcoal doses Alkalization of the urine (goal of urine pH 7.5) with use of bicarbonate infusion Hemodialysis for: • Levels >100 mg/dL • Seizures • Refractive metabolic derangements • Severe electrolyte disturbances
Sulfonylureas	Hypoglycemia, profound and persistent, depending on the formulation (sustained release) A single tablet of any of the sulfonylureas can result in significant toxicity Management Labs: even without symptoms, check glucose hourly Dextrose Volume: Do NOT use dextrose containing fluids UNLESS patient becomes hypoglycemic, due to masking onset of symptoms Hypoglycemia: 4 mL/kg D 10 via peripheral IV (D25 too caustic for most peripheral lines) Dextrose containing solutions, from D5 to D20 to keep serum glc >100	**Antidote:** Octreotide (inhibits pancreatic insulin secretion) *compliments* dextrose infusion. Dose: 4–5 µg/kg SQ *divided* every 6 h until can maintain blood glucose without IV dextrose (max dose 50 µg)

Antidotes

Indication	Antidote	*Initial* dose (peds dosing)
Acetaminophen	N-acetylcysteine	150 mg/kg IV over 1 h, then 50 mg/kg IV × 1 over 4 h, then 100 mg/kg IV × 1 over 16 h; requires special dilution in peds
Iron	Deferoxamine	Start IV infusion at 5 mg/kg/h; titrate up to 15 mg/kg/h, up to total of 6–8 gm/day
Digoxin	Dig-specific antibody	# vials IV = [dig level (ng/mL) × wt (kg)]/100
Methanol/ethylene glycol	Fomepizole	15 mg/kg, diluted in 100 mL over 30 min
Beta-blockers/Ca++ channel blockers	Glucagon	50 μg/kg given over 1–2 min (max dose 10 mg)
Methemoglobinemia	Methylene blue	0.1–0.2 mL/kg IV over 5 min (max dose 7 mg/kg)
Opioid, clonidine, Lomotil	Naloxone	0.1 mg/kg
Sulfonylureas	Octreotide	1.25 μg/kg SQ (max dose 50 μg)
Carbamates/organophosphates	Atropine (carbamates only); pralidoxime + atropine (organophosphates)	Atropine: 20 μg/kg Pralidoxime: 30 mg/kg infused over 15–30 min (pralidoxime) (max dose 2 g)
Isoniazid	Pyridoxine	70 mg/kg (max dose 5 g)

Acronyms

ACRONYMS

Causes of elevated anion gap: MUDPILES

M	Methanol, metformin
U	Uremia
D	Diabetic ketoacidosis
P	Paraldehyde, phenformin, phenothiazines
I	INH, iron
L	Lactic acidosis
E	Ethylene glycol, ETOH
S	Salicylates

Symptoms of cholinergic crisis: SLUDGE

S	Salivation
L	Lacrimation
U	Urination
D	Diaphoresis
G	Gastric distress (vomiting, diarrhea, cramping, abdominal pain)
E	Edema (bronchorrhea)

Causes of bradycardia: PACED

P	Propranolol
A	Anticholinesterase intoxicants (organophosphates), antiarrhythmics (Ca++ channel blockers and beta blockers)
C	Clonidine
E	Ethanol/other alcohols
D	Digoxin

Radiopaque: COINS

C	Chloral hydrate, cocaine packets, calcium
O	Opium packets
I	Iron and other heavy metals (lead, arsenic, mercury
N	Neuroleptic agents
S	Sustained release or enteric coated tablets (tendency to form bezoars)

Dialyzable Toxins: I STUMBLE

I	Isopropyl
S	Salicylates
T	Theophylline
U	Uremia
M	Methanol
B	Barbituates
L	Lithium
E	Ethylene glycol, ETOH

Activated Charcoal

Activated charcoal has not been proven to change the clinical outcome of ingested poisonings but can decrease serum drug levels if given within 1 h of ingestion.

Single dose	Multiple dose	Activated charcoal does NOT BIND:
• Give within 1st hour of ingestion • 1 g/kg • Max 50 g/dose	• Massive ingestions of toxicants known to be absorbed by activated charcoal • Suspected bezoar formation • Enteric coated or prolonged release formulation • Aspirin • Phenobarbital • Theophylline	• Corrosives (strong acids or bases) • Lithium • Arsenic • Alcohols • Inorganic minerals (sodium, iodine, fluorine) • Iron • Lead • Cyanide

Ingestions with Delayed Presentation

- Acetaminophen: Without symptoms for first 6–24 h (except in massive OD)
- Iron: Initial symptoms of GI distress (due to localized toxic effects on GI tract) abate, and second stage is "latent", or relatively asymptomatic.
- Mushrooms

    - *Amanita phalloides* (Deadly nightshade): 24 h (hepatic)
    - *Cortinarius* species—24 h (renal)

Useful Formulas

$$\text{Anion gap}(nL<15): Na^+ - \left(Cl^- + HCO3^-\right)$$

$$\text{Osmolar gap}(nL<10): \text{Measured serum osm} - \text{calculated osm}$$

$$\text{Calculated osm}: \left(2 \times Na\right) + \left(glc/18\right) + \left(BUN/2.8\right)$$

Button Battery Ingestion

- The 3 Ns (the negative battery pole, identified by the narrowest side on the lateral X-ray causes severe, necrotic injury).

  - Negative
  - Narrow
  - Necrotic

- 20 mm lithium cell battery is the most common cause of esophageal injuries.
- Hearing aid batteries are <12 mm.
- ANY button battery can cause severe, life threatening injury.
- Do not induce vomiting or give cathartics.
- Must perform X-rays of neck, chest, and abdomen so that batteries are not missed.
- Must obtain AP and lateral X-rays to determine orientation of the negative pole.
- If button battery ingestion is suspected and no battery is seen on X-ray, check the ears and nose.

Button Battery Ingestion Algorithm (Fig. 18.1)

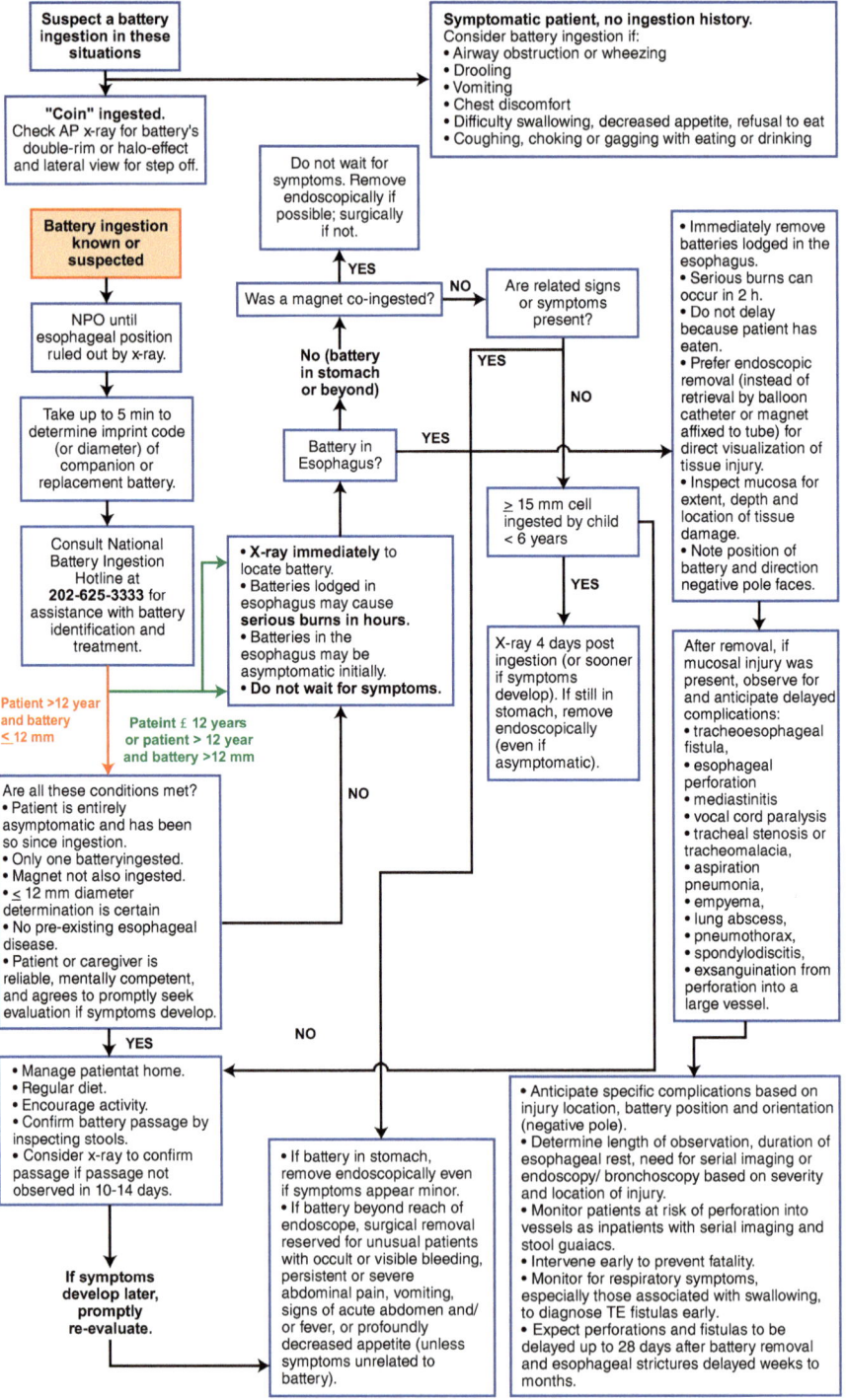

Fig. 18.1 Button battery ingestion algorithm

Chapter 19
Pediatric Pain

Cristina M. Zeretzke-Bien

Abstract The inappropriate dosing and poor recognition of pain in the pediatric patient are common pitfalls for ED providers. This chapter focuses on both pharmaceutical and distraction/integrative therapy to help you achieve appropriate analgesia before performing that next laceration repair or lumbar puncture.

Pediatric Pain

- Pain is one of the top reasons patients present to the emergency department!
- Pain is a *unique* experience to each patient.
- It is varied and is a different experience based on developmental age, prior experience, culture, gender, ethnicity, as well as patient expectations.
- It is important to address a *patient's pain* as it relates to the developmental age; if pain and anxiety can be managed, the provider and patient will have a much better outcome.
- A pain memory starts as early as 6 months!

Avoid Medication Errors

- Include generic drug name, dose (stated as mg/kg = total dose mg) frequency, rate, and route.

C. M. Zeretzke-Bien (✉)
Division of Pediatric Emergency Medicine, University of Florida, Gainesville, FL, USA
e-mail: Zeretzke@ufl.edu

© The Author(s), under exclusive license to Springer Nature
Switzerland AG 2023
C. M. Zeretzke-Bien, T. B. Swan (eds.), *Quick Hits for Pediatric Emergency Medicine*, https://doi.org/10.1007/978-3-031-32650-9_19

- Spell out micrograms to avoid transcription error.
- Spell out morphine to avoid medication error when writing "ms."
- Avoid decimal errors: write "1" not "1.0" which can cause tenfold dosing errors.

WHO Principles of Pain Management

- Apply the WHO pain ladder: DO NOT undermedicate. Advance to opioids if pain control is suboptimal.
- Use around-the-clock pain medications if predictable PLUS additional pain medications for BREAKTHROUGH pain doses.
- Use the simplest and least invasive when possible (oral vs. intranasal vs. IV).
- Assess the pain regularly and change the plan accordingly.
- Use combinations of non-opioids and an opioid to enhance pain control.
- Always integrate NON-DRUG strategies in combination with medications to enhance pain control.

Infant FLACC Scale

Scoring

Numeric Scale

Use 0 (no pain) to 10 (worst pain you can imagine) scale for children older than 7 years of age (Fig. 19.1)

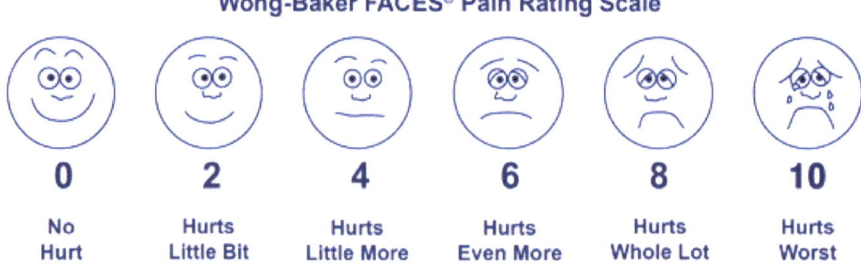

Fig. 19.1 Wong-Baker Faces Pain Scale

Topical Local Anesthetics

Should always be offered!

- LMX (LMX 4% topical anesthetic cream contains 4% lidocaine and can be used to relieve pain) (at least 30 min).
- EMLA (a mixture of lidocaine 2.5% and prilocaine 2.5%) is indicated as a topical anesthetic for use on normal intact skin for local analgesia (60 min).
- J-tip (needleless lidocaine injector) consider with all IV starts.

Non-pharmaceutical Methods

Distraction and Integrative Therapies

Types of Distraction

1. Passive distraction: attention is redirected to a stimulus or an object.

   (a) Showing a toy, storytelling, singing songs, or playing with pinwheels.

2. Active distraction: encourage participation in activities during procedures.

   (b) Blowing bubbles, playing a game, or interacting with an electronic device.

Other Integrative Therapies

- Relaxation techniques (diaphragmatic breathing)
- Guided imagery
- Music therapy
- Ice pack or warm pack
- Hypnosis
- Tablet/smartphone

Sucrose (0–12 Months)

- Reduces cry and pain during painful procedures, such as venipuncture.
- Effective dose (24%) 0.05–0.5 mL (=0.012–0.12 g)
- Administer 2 min prior to mild/moderately painful procedures
- Duration is approximately 4 min.

Pharmacological Treatment of Pain

Non-opioids commonly sed for mild to moderate pain.
  Opioid analgesics used for moderate to severe pain.
  Opioid analgesics used for moderate to severe pain (IV form).

Opioid Antagonist

Sedation: Consider sedation when analgesia not feasible, minimal, or moderate/deep sedation.

Procedural anxiety: Midazolam (Versed) (5 mg/mL), 0.3–0.4 mg/kg. Max dose, 10 mg or 1 mL per nostril (total 2 mL) (use with atomizer if possible); divide each dose between each nostril.

Quick Hits Painful Procedure Pearls

1. Consider child life if available OR use parent/caregiver as "comfort coach."
2. Comfort positioning: Will increase sense of support and decrease resistance to the procedure.
3. When feasible offer a parent's lap. Do not lay child supine unless necessary.
4. Consider topical medications prior to procedure (with oral pain meds).
5. Use a tiny needle (25 gauge)—Draw up medications with a separate needle (out of sight of child).
6. Inject with the smallest needle. Slow and steady injection.
7. At the time of injection, rub or stroke the skin near the injection site.
8. Buffer lidocaine prior to injection.

Adapted from PAMI (Pain Assessment and Management Initiative) available at http://pami.emergency.med.jax.ufl.edu and from Pediatric Acute Pain Management Reference Card, Children's Hospitals and Clinic of Minnesota.

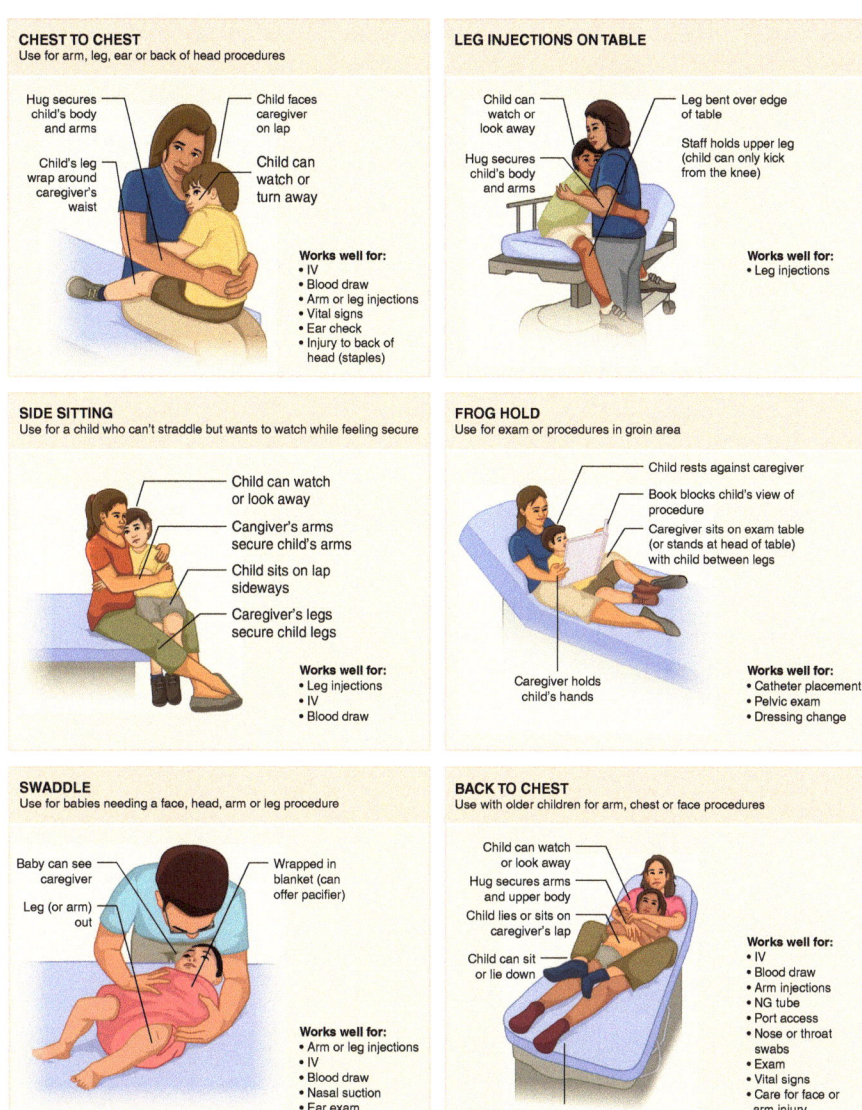

Comfort Hold

Chapter 20
Pediatric Antibiotic Guide

Tricia B. Swan and Vanessa Perez

Abstract This is a must-have guide to antibiotic therapy with both disease-specific suggested treatment as well as a quick guide to common pediatric antibiotics and their dosages. Truly a "Quick Hit" for antibiotics to keep you efficient while keeping your patient safe. The chapter even concludes with a table illustrating the bacterial coverage of the most commonly used antibiotics to ensure adequate antibacterial coverage as indicated.

T. B. Swan
Division of Pediatric Emergency Medicine, University of Florida, Gainesville, FL, USA
e-mail: tfalgiani@ufl.edu

V. Perez (✉)
Division of Pediatric Emergency Medicine, Nemours Children's Health, Orlando, FL, USA

University of Central Florida College of Medicine, Orlando, FL, USA
e-mail: vanessa.perez@nemours.org

C. M. Zeretzke-Bien, T. B. Swan (eds.), *Quick Hits for Pediatric Emergency Medicine*, https://doi.org/10.1007/978-3-031-32650-9_20

Infection	Common etiologies	Suggested therapy	Special considerations and length of treatment
Bites			
Human	*Streptococcus* spp., *Staphylococcus* spp., *Eikenella corrodens*, oral anaerobes, *Haemophilus* spp.	**PO:** Amoxicillin/clavulanate Alt: Clindamycin + (TMP/SMX *or* third generation cephalosporin) **IV:** Ampicillin/sulbactam Alt: TMP/SMX + clindamycin	Treatment for 5–7 days Ensure cleaning, copious irrigation, and debridement of wound Do not suture puncture wounds Assess Hep B and tetanus immunization status Evaluate HIV risk
Dog, cat, or mammal	*Pasteurella* species, *Staphylococcus aureus*, streptococci, *Capnocytophaga* species, *Moraxella* species, *Corynebacterium* species	Same as above	Treatment for 7–10 days Ensure cleaning, copious irrigation, and debridement of wound Do not suture puncture wounds Assess tetanus immunization status Assess rabies risk and provide rabies immunoglobulin (RIG) + rabies vaccine if indicated
Cellulitis/skin abscess	*S. aureus* (MSSA or MRSA), *Streptococcus pyogenes*	**PO:** Cephalexin or clindamycin if MRSA suspected **IV:** Oxacillin; clindamycin, or vancomycin if MRSA suspected TMP/SMX is not active against group A *streptococcus*	Treatment for 5–7 days Incision and drainage should be performed if abscess is present Hospitalize for severe infections, immunocompromised state or limb threatening infections
Conjunctivitis (non-neonatal)	*S. Pneumonia, H. influenza, Moraxella*, viral	Erythromycin ophthalmic ointment, bacitracin/polymyxin B, or polymyxin B/TMP drops Levofloxacin solution for contact lens wearers	Treatment for 5 days Most conjunctivitis is viral in etiology, but CDC recommends topical antibiotic treatment when purulent exudate is present

Conjunctivitis (neonatal)	*N. gonorrhoeae*	Ceftriaxone or cefotaxime	Onset 2–5 days of age Single dose IV/IM Admit for evaluation and treatment of possible disseminated disease
	C. Trachomatis	Azithromycin for 5 days or erythromycin for 14 days	Onset 5–12 days of age
Dacryocystitis	*S. pneumoniae, H. influenzae, S. aureus, S. pyogenes, Pseudomonas aeruginosa*	Oxacillin or cephalexin	Treatment for 7–10 days Warm compresses
Dental abscess	Oral floral, anaerobes	Amoxicillin/clavulanate or clindamycin	Treatment for 10 days Refer for dental evaluation and surgical drainage
Intra-abdominal infection	*E. coli, Enterococcus, Bacteroides* spp., *Clostridium* spp., *P. aeruginosa, S. aureus, Klebsiella* species (often polymicrobial)	*Mild to moderate:* Ceftriaxone PLUS Metronidazole *Severe or hospital onset:* Piperacillin-tazobactam OR Ciprofloxacin PLUS Metronidazole	Treatment 5–7 days Consider MRSA coverage in patients concerning for health care-associated infections
Lymphadenitis	Viruses, group A *Strep.*, *S. aureus, Actinomyces*, anaerobes, atypical mycobacteria, *Mycobacterium tuberculosis*, *Bartonella* species (cat scratch disease)	**PO:** Amoxicillin/clavulanate; clindamycin if MRSA suspected Azithromycin for cat scratch Alt: Dicloxacillin or cephalexin **IV:** Oxacillin or cefazolin; clindamycin if MRSA suspected	Treatment for 7 days If PCN allergic may use cefdinir, cefuroxime, or clindamycin Bacterial adenitis is typically unilateral; bilateral disease is typically viral in etiology
Mastoiditis	*Streptococcus pneumoniae, S. pyogenes, S. aureus, Hemophilus influenzae* Consider MRSA based on local prevalence	**PO:** Amoxicillin/clavulanate or third generation cephalosporin **IV:** Ampicillin-sulbactam OR Ceftriaxone *If follows chronic AOM:* Cefepime OR Levofloxacin	Patients with mild mastoiditis may be treated as outpatient with oral antibiotics Treatment up to 4 weeks May require surgical drainage Ampicillin-sulbactam may not be optimal if intracranial extension

Infection	Common etiologies	Suggested therapy	Special considerations and length of treatment
Meningitis (neonatal)	Group B streptococcus (GBS), *E. coli*, *Listeria monocytogenes*, HSV	*Neonates 0–7 days:* Ampicillin PLUS Gentamicin *Neonates 8–28 days:* Ampicillin PLUS Cefotaxime (Ceftazidime or Cefepime if Cefotaxime is not available) Consider adding acyclovir with surface, blood, and CSF HSV sampling	Treatment for 14 days for GBS, 21 days for *Listeria* and *E. coli* Gentamicin is less preferred due to poor CSF penetration
Meningitis (>1 month of age)	*S. pneumoniae, H. influenzae, N. meningitidis, E. coli*	IV: Ceftriaxone PLUS Vancomycin	Duration of treatment depends on organism
Orbital cellulitis (septal)	*S. pneumoniae, S. aureus, H. influenzae, M. catarrhalis*, group A streptococcus, anaerobes	IV: Vancomycin or clindamycin plus (ampicillin/sulbactam or ceftriaxone or cefotaxime)	Treatment for 10–14 days Needs ophthalmology consult CT head to evaluate for intracranial extension
Osteomyelitis	*S. aureus, Streptococcus* spp., group A streptococcus, *Kingella kingae* (<4 years of age) Foot puncture: *P. aeruginosa* Sickle cell disease: *Salmonella* spp.	Cefazolin, Oxacillin, Nafcillin, or Clindamycin Alt: TMP-SMX **Foot puncture**: Add ceftazidime or antipseudomonal penicillin **Sickle cell disease**: Add ceftriaxone	Treatment for 4–6 weeks Clindamycin monotherapy not effective for *Kingella*
Otitis media	*S. pneumoniae, H. influenzae, M. catarrhalis, S. pyogenes*, viral Consider *S. aureus* and *Pseudomonas* for chronic otitis media	Amoxicillin (90 mg/kg/day) Amoxicillin-clavulanate IF amoxicillin treatment in the last 30 days or concurrent purulent conjunctivitis **Treatment failure:** Amoxicillin-clavulanate OR Cefdinir, OR Ceftriaxone (1–3 days)	Treatment: >6 years: 5 days 2–5 years: 7 days <2 years or severe symptoms: 10 days Definition of treatment failure: Fever, bulging TM, no change in ear pain or otorrhea after 3 days of treatment
Otitis externa	*Staphylococcus* spp., *P. aeruginosa, Bacteroides* spp.	Otic solution: Ciprofloxacin, ciprofloxacin/dexamethasone, ofloxacin, or polymyxin B/neomycin/hydrocortisone	Treatment for 7–10 days Consider cerumen removal to expedite resolution

Condition	Organisms	Treatment	Comments
Parotitis	*S. aureus* most common, oral flora, gram negative rods, viral (mumps, HIV, EBV, parainfluenza), and non-infectious causes	**PO:** Clindamycin or Amoxicillin-clavulanate **IV:** Cefazolin, Nafcillin Clindamycin	Treatment for 10–14 days Establish duct patency with warm compresses, sialagogues, gentle massage of gland and hydration Surgical drainage may be required
Periorbital cellulitis (pre-septal)	*S. pneumoniae, S. aureus, H. influenzae, M. catarrhalis,* group A streptococcus, anaerobes	**PO:** Amoxicillin/clavulanate or third generation cephalosporin **IV:** Ampicillin/sulbactam If concerned for MRSA add TMP/SMX, clindamycin, or vancomycin	Treatment for 10–14 days CT scan of orbits helps to differentiate from orbital cellulitis Indications for CT: Proptosis, ophthalmoplegia, change in visual acuity, bilateral periorbital edema, inability to assess vision secondary to edema, no improvement after 24 h of outpatient therapy
Pertussis	*Bordetella pertussis*	Azithromycin or erythromycin Use azithromycin in children <1 month	Treatment for 5 days with azithromycin or 7–14 days with erythromycin Chemoprophylaxis for close contacts
Pharyngitis	Group A, C, and G streptococci, *Arcanobacterium haemolyticum,* viral (EBV, coxsackievirus, others)	**PO:** Amoxicillin or PCN V **IM:** Penicillin G benzathine ×1 If PCN allergy: Clindamycin, Cephalexin, or oral macrolides	Treatment must be full 10 days to prevent acute rheumatic fever in GAS infections Supportive treatment for viral pharyngitis
Pneumonia (community acquired)			
Age < 5 years	*S. pneumoniae, H. influenzae, Mycoplasma,* group A streptococcus, *C. pneumoniae, S. aureus,* viral (Influenza, SARS-COVID-2, RSV)	**PO:** High dose Amoxicillin ± Azithromycin (atypical coverage) Alt: Clindamycin, Amoxicillin-clavulanate, Cefdinir **IV:** Ampicillin ± Azithromycin Alt: Ceftriaxone ± Azithromycin Add Vancomycin or Clindamycin if sepsis, severe illness or features suggestive of *S. aureus* (cavitation, pleural effusion)	Treatment for 10 days Respiratory viruses cause the majority of CAP in young children

Infection	Common etiologies	Suggested therapy	Special considerations and length of treatment
Age > 5 years and immunized	S. pneumoniae, Mycoplasma, group A streptococcus, C. pneumoniae, S. aureus, viral (influenza, SARS-COVID-2)	**PO:** High dose Amoxicillin PLUS Azithromycin (atypical coverage) Alt: Clindamycin PLUS Azithromycin **IV:** Ampicillin PLUS Azithromycin Alt: Ceftriaxone PLUS Azithromycin Add Vancomycin or Clindamycin if sepsis, severe illness or features suggestive of S. aureus (cavitation, pleural effusion)	Treatment for 7–10 days Atypical organisms (Mycoplasma, Chlamydia) are more common in children >5 years old Consider S. aureus superinfection in patients with influenza
Age > 5 years and unimmunized for H. influenzae or S. pneumoniae	S. pneumoniae, Mycoplasma, group A streptococcus, C. pneumoniae, S. aureus, viral, influenza	Ceftriaxone ± Azithromycin Add Vancomycin or Clindamycin if severe illness or features suggestive of S. aureus (cavitation, pleural effusion)	Treatment for 10 days
Retropharyngeal abscess	S. aureus, S. pyogenes, anaerobes, Streptococcus anginosus, H. influenzae (often polymicrobial)	*Mild to moderate:* Ampicillin-sulbactam OR clindamycin *Severe:* Ampicillin-sulbactam PLUS EITHER Vancomycin OR linezolid	Treatment for 14 days
Septic arthritis			
Age < 5 years	S. aureus, S. pyogenes, S. pneumoniae, Kingella kingae	Cefazolin OR Oxacillin OR Clindamycin Add Amoxicillin for Kingella *Severe infection:* Vancomycin PLUS EITHER Cefazolin, OR Oxacillin OR Nafcillin	Treatment for 2–3 weeks Aspiration of affected joint recommended Joint aspirate >50,000 WBC with PMN predominance is associated with septic arthritis (although 33% will have less)
Age > 5 years	S. aureus, group A streptococcus, Streptococcus spp.	Clindamycin or vancomycin plus (ceftriaxone or cefotaxime)	Treatment for 2–3 weeks Aspiration of affected joint recommended Joint aspirate >50,000 WBC with PMN predominance is associated with septic arthritis (although 33% will have less)

Adolescent	Add *N. gonorrhoeae*	Add Ceftriaxone	Treatment for 3 weeks (IV) Aspiration of affected joint recommended Consider gonococcal infection in polyarticular arthritis All patients with suspected gonococcal infection should also be treated with Doxycycline or Azithromycin to cover possible concurrent *C. trachomatis* infection
Sexually transmitted infections			
Urethritis and cervicitis Bacterial vaginosis	*N. gonorrhoeae, C. trachomatis* *T. vaginalis*	Ceftriaxone IM once AND Doxycycline for 10 days Metronidazole	
Sinusitis			
Acute	*S. pneumoniae, S. aureus, H. influenzae, M. catarrhalis*	Amoxicillin-clavulanate If PCN allergy: Clindamycin OR Levofloxacin	For acute uncomplicated bacterial sinusitis and reliable follow-up consider watchful waiting and defer antibiotic therapy and treat with intra-nasal saline rinses and intra-nasal corticosteroids **Indication for antibiotic treatment**: No improvement in 10 days, fever >39 °C, and purulent nasal drainage, facial pain >3 days, worsening symptoms following viral URI for 6 days that was initially improving Treatment for 10–14 days If no improvement in 3–5 days, broaden coverage Severe symptoms or failure to respond: Consider imaging and drainage **Warning:** The use of fluoroquinolones should be reserved for patients when there is no other therapeutic alternative

Infection	Common etiologies	Suggested therapy	Special considerations and length of treatment
Chronic	Add S. aureus, anaerobes	Amoxicillin-clavulanate, Cefpodoxime, Cefuroxime OR Cefdinir Alt: Fluoroquinolone	Treat for 7 additional days after resolution of symptoms See above **Warning:** The use of fluoroquinolones should be reserved for patients when there is no other therapeutic alternative
Seriously ill or immunocompromised	Add Pseudomonas, gram-negative bacilli, Mucor, Rhizopus, and Aspergillus coverage	Cefepime or Piperacillin/tazobactam + Amphotericin B	Surgical intervention needed See above
Tracheitis	S. aureus, S. pneumoniae, M. catarrhalis, H. influenzae, Pseudomonas, group A streptococcus	Community acquired: Ceftriaxone plus clindamycin Ventilator or tracheostomy dependent: Cefepime or Piperacillin/tazobactam	Treatment for 7–10 days
UTI			
Cystitis	E. coli, Proteus Spp., Enterobacteriaceae, Staphylococcus saprophyticus, Enterococcus spp.	**PO:** Cephalexin OR TMP-SMX **IV:** Ampicillin PLUS Gentamicin OR Ceftriaxone Alt: Nitrofurantoin or Ciprofloxacin	Treatment for 3–5 days (simple cystitis in adolescents), 7–10 days (febrile UTI depending on response) **Warning:** The use of fluoroquinolones should be reserved for patients when there is no other therapeutic alternative
Pyelonephritis	E. coli, Proteus Spp., Enterobacteriaceae, Enterococcus spp.	Ceftriaxone OR Ampicillin PLUS Gentamycin Alt: Cefdinir or Ciprofloxacin	Treatment 7–14 days (TID) **Warning:** The use of fluoroquinolones should be reserved for patients when there is no other therapeutic alternative
Abnormal host/urinary tract	Add Pseudomonas, resistant gram-negative organisms	Piperacillin/tazobactam or cefepime	Treatment for 7–14 days

Common Pediatric Antibiotic Drugs and Dosages

Drug	Dose	Coverage	Common uses	Special considerations
Amoxicillin	**Standard dose:** 40–50 mg/kg/day ÷ Q 8–12 h PO **High dose:** 80–90 mg/kg/day ÷ Q 8–12 h PO Max dose: 2–3 g/day	*S. pneumoniae, H. influenzae, S. pyogenes, S. aureus, M. catarrhalis*	Acute otitis media, Community acquired pneumonia, strep pharyngitis	• Adjust dose in renal failure • High dose regimen is increasingly useful and recommended in respiratory infection and acute otitis media • GI side effects common
Amoxicillin-clavulanate	80–90 mg/kg/day ÷ Q 8–12 h PO	*S. pneumoniae, H. influenzae, S. pyogenes, S. aureus, M. catarrhalis, N. gonorrhoeae,* some *S. aureus*	Acute otitis media, community acquired pneumonia, sinusitis, animal and human bites	• Adjust dose in renal failure • GI side effects common
Ampicillin	**Group B streptococcal meningitis (GBS):** ≤7 days: 200–300 mg/kg/day ÷ Q 8 h IV ≥7 days: 300 mg/kg/day ÷ Q 6 h IV **Infant/child:** **Mild/moderate infections:** 100–200 mg/kg/day ÷ Q 6 h IV/IM 50–100 mg/kg/day ÷ Q 6 h PO **Severe infections:** 200–400 mg/kg/day ÷ Q 4–6 h IV/IM Max PO dose: 2-g/day Max IV/IM dose: 12 g/day	*L. monocytogenes, S. pneumoniae, S. pyogenes* (GBS), some *S. aureus,* some *Enterococcus, N. meningitidis, H. influenzae,* some Enterobacteriaceae	Meningitis, pneumonia, otitis media, urinary tract infection, salmonellosis, endocarditis	• Use higher dose with shorter dosing intervals in patients with CNS disease or severe infection • Adjust dose in renal failure • GI side effects common

Drug	Dose	Coverage	Common uses	Special considerations
Azithromycin	**Child:** 10 mg/kg once daily on day 1, then 5 mg/kg once daily on days 2–5 **Adolescent/adult:** 500 mg/day once daily on day 1, then 250 mg/day once daily on days 2–5 **Pharyngitis:** 12 mg/kg/day once daily for 5 days **Chlamydial cervicitis/ urethritis:** 1 g PO×1 **Gonococcal cervicitis/ urethritis:** 2 g PO × 1 **Acute PID:** 500 mg IV × 1 on day 1, then 250 mg once daily for 6 days Max dose 500 mg/day (except in cervicitis/PID treatment)	*H. influenzae, M. catarrhalis, S. pneumoniae, S. aureus, S. pyogenes, S. agalactiae, C. trachomatis and pneumoniae, N. gonorrhoeae, B. pertussis, Legionella pneumophila, M. pneumoniae*	Pneumonia, pertussis, pharyngitis, sinusitis, chlamydial/gonococcal cervicitis/urethritis/PID, atypical infections, otitis media (alternative therapy), uncomplicated skin infections, traveler's diarrhea	• Absorbed best on an empty stomach • Use with caution in patients with arrhythmias or prolonged QT interval • IV administration over 1–3 h • GI side effects common
Cefazolin (first generation)	50–100 mg/kg/day ÷ Q 6–8 h IV/IM (>1 month of age) Max dose 6 g/day	*S. aureus, S. epidermidis, S. pyogenes, S. agalactiae, S. pneumoniae, E.coli, Proteus mirabilis*	Cellulitis, UTI, endocarditis, biliary tract infections, surgical prophylaxis	• Does not penetrate CSF • Dosing adjustment required for children <1 month of age • Adjust dose for renal failure
Cefdinir (third generation)	14 mg/kg/day ÷ Q 12–24 h PO Max dose 600 mg/day	*S. aureus, H. influenzae, S. pneumoniae, S. pyogenes, M. catarrhalis*	Otitis media, pharyngitis, sinusitis, skin infections, community acquired pneumonia, UTI	• May cause red- or orange-colored stools • BID dosing is recommended over once daily dosing • Adjust dose for renal failure

	Dosing	Spectrum	Indications	Comments
Cefepime (fourth generation)	Children ≥2 months: 100 mg/kg/day ÷ Q 12 h IV/IM Meningitis/fever with neutropenia/serious infection/cystic fibrosis: 150 mg/kg/day ÷ Q 8 h IV/IM Max dose: 6 g/day	Broad spectrum against gram positive and gram-negative organisms + *Pseudomonas aeruginosa*	Meningitis, fever in neutropenic patients, cystic fibrosis patients, tracheitis with pseudomonas infection, severe illness	• Dosing adjustment required for children <1 month of age • Adjust dose for renal failure
Cefotaxime (third generation)	**Neonate (IV/IM):** **≤7 days old:** <2 kg: 100 mg/kg/day ÷ Q 12 h ≥2 kg: 100–150 mg/kg/day ÷ Q 8 h **>7 days old:** <1.2 kg: 100 mg/kg/day ÷ Q 12 h 1.2–2 kg: 150 mg/kg/day ÷ Q 8 h >2 kg: 150–200 mg/kg/day ÷ Q 6–8 h **Infant and children:** 100–200 mg/kg/day ÷ Q 6 h (use 200 mg/kg/day for meningitis dosing) Max dose: 12 g/day	*S. aureus, S. epidermidis, S. pyogenes, S. agalactiae, S. pneumoniae, S. epidermidis, E. coli, Proteus mirabilis, N. meningitidis, H. influenzae, Neisseria gonorrhoeae, Klebsiella spp., Burkholderia cepacia, Enterobacter spp., Bacteroides spp., Fusobacterium spp.*	Neonatal meningitis, meningitis, pneumonia, severe infections, skin infections, gonorrhea, PID	• Adjust dose for renal failure

Drug	Dose	Coverage	Common uses	Special considerations
Cefotetan (second generation)	40–80 mg/kg/day ÷ Q 12 h IV/IM Adolescent/adult: 2–4 g/day ÷ Q 12 h IV/IM Max dose 6 g/day	Some gram-positive coverage, good gram-negative coverage, *Bacteroides* spp.. *Streptococcus* spp., and *Escherichia* spp.	Uncomplicated skin infections, PID, UTI, pharyngitis, preoperative prophylaxis	• Good anaerobic activity • Poor CSF penetration. Adjust dose for renal failure
Cefprozil (second generation)	30 mg/kg/day ÷ Q 12 h PO Pharyngitis: 15 mg/kg/day ÷ Q 12 h PO Max dose 1 g/day	Some gram-positive coverage, good gram-negative coverage, *Bacteroides* spp.. *Streptococcus* spp., and *Escherichia* spp.	Uncomplicated skin infections, PID, UTI, sinusitis, otitis media, pharyngitis, preoperative prophylaxis	• Adjust dose for renal failure
Ceftazidime (third generation)	**Neonate (IV/IM):** **≤7 days old:** <2 kg: 100 mg/kg/day ÷ Q 12 h ≥2 kg: 100–150 mg/kg/day ÷ Q 8–12 h **>7 days old:** <1.2 kg: 100 mg/kg/day ÷ Q 12 h >1.2 kg: 150 mg/kg/day ÷ Q 8 h **Infant and children (IV/IM):** 100–150 mg/kg/day ÷ Q 8 h Max dose: 6 g/day	*Enterobacter, E. coli, H. influenzae, Klebsiella, Proteus, Pseudomonas, N. meningitidis, Neisseria gonorrhoeae,* group B streptococci, *S. pneumoniae,* and *S. pyogenes, Bacteroides*	Meningitis, cystic fibrosis patients, pneumonia, sepsis, UTI, joint infections	• Adjust dose for renal failure

| Ceftriaxone (third generation) | **Gonococcal ophthalmia (IV/IM):** 25–50 mg/kg/dose × 1 dose (max dose 125 mg/dose) **Infants (>1 month) and children (IV/IM):** Mild/moderate infection: 50–75 mg/kg/day ÷ Q 12–24 h Meningitis: 100 mg/kg/day ÷ Q 12 h Uncomplicated gonorrhea: 500 mg IM × 1 dose; if >150 kg 1 g IM × 1 Max dose: 2 g/dose and 4 g/day | *Staphylococcus* spp., *E. coli, H. influenzae, Klebsiella, Proteus* spp., *N. meningitidis,* group B streptococci, *S. pneumoniae,* and *S. pyogenes, Bacteroides* | Meningitis, pneumonia, otitis media, sinusitis, gonococcal ophthalmia, gonorrhea, PID, UTI, bone and joint infections, intra-abdominal infections, uncomplicated skin infections, endocarditis, sepsis | • Unlike other cephalosporins, ceftriaxone is significantly cleared by the biliary route, therefore is contraindicated in neonates with hyperbilirubinemia
• Particularly those who are premature because ceftriaxone may displace bilirubin from albumin binding sites, causing bilirubin encephalopathy
• No activity against *Chlamydia trachomatis*
• **Concomitant use with intravenous calcium-containing solutions/products is contraindicated** |
| Cephalexin (first generation) | 25–100 mg/kg/day ÷ Q 6–12 h PO Streptococcal pharyngitis: 25–50 mg/kg/day ÷ Q 6–12 h PO Max dose 4 g/day | *S. aureus, S. pyogenes, S. pneumoniae, H. influenzae, E. coli, Proteus mirabilis, Klebsiella pneumoniae* | Uncomplicated skin infections, pharyngitis, UTI, pyelonephritis, bone, and joint infections | • Less frequent dosing (Q 12 h) may be used for uncomplicated infections |

Drug	Dose	Coverage	Common uses	Special considerations
Clindamycin	**Neonate (IV/IM):** **<7 days old:** <2 kg: 5 mg/kg/day ÷ Q 12 h ≥2 kg: 5 mg/kg/day ÷ Q 8 h **>7 days old:** <1.2 kg: 5 mg/kg/day ÷ Q 12 h 1.2–2 kg: 5 mg/kg/day ÷ Q 8 h >2 kg: 5 mg/kg/day ÷ Q 6 h **Child:** **PO:** 10–30 mg/kg/day ÷ Q 6–8 h **IV/IM:** 25–40 mg/kg/day ÷ Q 6–8 h **Adult:** **PO:** 150–450 mg/dose Q 6–8 h **IV/IM:** 1200–1800 mg/day ÷ Q 6–12 h Max PO dose: 1.8 g/day Max IV/IM dose: 4.8 g/day	Methicillin-resistant *Staphylococcus aureus*, *Staphylococcus* spp., *Streptococcus* spp., *Bacteroides* spp., *Fusobacterium* spp., *Prevotella* spp.	Skin infections, skin abscess, MRSA infections, acne, otitis media, pneumonia, empyema, bone and joint infections, pharyngitis, PID	• Poor CSF penetration • Oral liquid not palatable, consider oral capsules, and sprinkle into pudding or applesauce • Serious side effects include pseudomembranous colitis, Steven-Johnson syndrome, thrombocytopenia, granulocytopenia
Gentamicin	**Neonates/infants:** 4 mg/kg/day ÷ Q 12–48 h **(dosing intervals vary for neonates based on gestational age, please refer to trusted resource)** **Child:** 7.5 mg/kg/day ÷ Q 8 h **Adult:** 3–6 mg/kg/day ÷ Q 8 h	Gram-negative bacteria including *Pseudomonas*, *Proteus* spp., *Escherichia coli*, *Klebsiella pneumoniae*, *Enterobacter aerogenes*, *Serratia* spp., and the Gram-positive *Staphylococcus*	Neonatal meningitis, neonatal sepsis, meningitis, bone infections, endocarditis, pneumonia, urinary tract infections, sepsis	• May be ototoxic and nephrotoxic • Adjust dose in renal failure

Piperacillin/tazobactam	**Neonate:** **<1 kg:** 100 mg/kg/dose Q 12 h (0–14 days old) or Q 8 h (15–28 days old) **>1 kg:** 100 mg/kg/dose Q 12 h (0–7 days old) or Q 8 h (8–28 days old) **Severe infections:** **<2 months:** 300–400 mg/kg/day ÷ Q 6 h **2–9 months:** 240 mg/kg/day ÷ Q 8 h **>9 months:** 300 mg/kg/day ÷ Q 8 h Max dose 16 g/day	*S. aureus, E. coli, Haemophilus influenzae, B. fragilis, B. ovatus, B. thetaiotaomicron, B. vulgatus. Klebsiella pneumoniae,* and *Pseudomonas aeruginosa*	Intra-abdominal infections, skin infections, pneumonia, severe infections, peritonitis	• Shortening dosing interval to Q 6 h may enhance pharmacodynamics properties • CSF penetration occurs only with inflamed meninges
Sulfamethoxazole/trimethoprim	**Dosed based on TMP component:** **Mild–moderated infections (PO or IV):** <40 kg: 8–12 mg/kg/day ÷ Q 12 h >40 kg: 160 mg/dose BID **Severe infections (PO or IV):** 20 g/kg/day ÷ Q 6–8 h	Methicillin-resistant *Staphylococcus aureus, Staphylococcus* spp., *Streptococcus* spp., *Bartonella henselae, Bordetella pertussis, Enterobacter* spp., *E. coli, H. influenzae, Listeria monocytogenes, Moraxella catarrhalis, Mycobacterium tuberculosis, Neisseria gonorrhoeae, Neisseria meningitidis, Pneumocystis jirovecii, Proteus* spp., *Salmonella* spp., *Shigella* spp., *Vibrio cholerae*	UTI, skin infections, skin abscess, MRSA skin infections, traveler's diarrhea, cholera, pneumocystis pneumonia in immunosuppressed patients	• Not recommended for use in infants <2 months of age • Serious side effects include blood dyscrasias, renal or hepatic injury, Stevens-Johnson syndrome • May cause hemolysis in patients with G6PD deficiency • Adjust dose for renal impairment

Drug	Dose	Coverage	Common uses	Special considerations
Vancomycin	**Neonate (IV): (dosing intervals vary for neonates based on gestational age, please refer to trusted resource)** Bacteremia: 10 mg/kg/dose Meningitis/pneumonia: 15 mg/kg/dose **Infant/child/adolescent (IV):** 15–20 mg/kg/day ÷ Q 6–8 h **Clostridium difficile colitis (PO):** Child: 40–50 mg/kg/day ÷ Q 6 h Adult: 125 mg/dose Q 6 h Max dose: 2 g/day	Methicillin-resistant *S. aureus* (MRSA), *C. difficile*, *Staphylococcus* spp., *Streptococcus* spp., some enterococci	Complicated skin infections, abscess, bacteremia, endocarditis, bone and joint infections, and meningitis caused by methicillin-resistant *S. aureus*, *Clostridium difficile* colitis	• Ototoxicity and nephrotoxicity may occur • Adjust dose in renal failure • Red man syndrome may occur with rapid IV infusion

Antibiotic	1	2	3	4	5	6
Penicillin	+	Limited	–	–	±	–
Oxacillin	+	–	–	–	–	–
Ampicillin	+	Limited	–	–	–	–
Amoxicillin	+	Limited	–	–	–	–
Amoxicillin/clavulanate (PO)	+	+	–	–	+	–
Ampicillin/sulbactam (IV)				–		
Piperacillin/tazobactam	+	+	+	–	+	–
Imipenem	+	+	+	+	–	–
Ciprofloxacin		+	+	–	–	+
Moxifloxacin	+	+	–	–	+	+
Levofloxacin	+	+	+	–		+
Cefazolin (first gen)	Limited	+	–	–	–	–
Cephalexin (first gen)	Limited	+	–	–	–	–
Cefoxitin (second gen)	Limited	+	–	–	+	–
Cefotetan (second gen)	Limited	+	–	–	+	–
Ceftriaxone (third gen)	+	+	–	–	–	–
Cefdinir (third gen)	+	+	–	–	–	–
Cefepime (fourth gen)	+	+	+	–	–	–
Gentamicin		+	+	–	–	–
Clindamycin	+	Limited	–	+	+	–
Vancomycin	+	–	–	+	–	–
Trimethoprim/sulfa	+	+	–	+	–	–
Tetracyclines	+	+	–	+	Limited	+
Linezolid	+	–	–	+	–	–
Metronidazole	–	–	–	–	+	–
Azithromycin	Limited	–	–	–	–	+

Quick Hits Pediatric Antibiotic Guide Pearls

1. Due to rapidly evolving resistance in organisms that cause common sexually transmitted infections (STIs), always check the Center for Disease (CDC) website for the most up-to-date outpatient and inpatient antibiotic regimens. https://www.cdc.gov/std/treatment-guidelines/toc.htm
2. Consider your local antibiogram when selecting antibiotics for specific disease conditions.
3. For acute otitis media associated with acute bacterial conjunctivitis, the first line therapy is amoxicillin-clavulanate (not amoxicillin).
4. Consider watchful waiting, rather than immediate antibiotic treatment, for patients older than 6 months of age with unilateral acute otitis media, mild otalgia, and temperature less than 39 °C *or* children older than 2 years of age with unilateral or bilateral AOM without otorrhea and mild symptoms.

When possible, obtain cultures with sensitivities of the infected site to help guide antibiotic management.

Chapter 21
Pediatric Diabetic Ketoacidosis

**Peyton Bennett, Cullen Clark, Anna McFarlin,
and Cristina M. Zeretzke-Bien**

Abstract This chapter on evaluation and management of diabetic ketoacidosis (DKA) allows the provider to be confident in their assessment and resuscitation of this potentially critically ill patient. The total fluid deficit equation and recommendations on rehydration are Quick Hits that will save lives.

Pediatric Diabetic Ketoacidosis

- *Definition*

  - Hyperglycemia: glucose >200
  - Metabolic acidosis pH <7.30 or HCO_3 <15
  - Ketosis: ketones in blood or urine

- *Signs and Symptoms*

  - Dehydration
  - Vomiting
  - Abdominal pain

P. Bennett
Pediatric Residency Program, Department of Pediatrics, Louisiana State University Health Science Center, New Orleans, LA, USA

C. Clark
Pediatrics and Emergency Medicine, The Ohio State University College of Medicine, Columbus, OH, USA

A. McFarlin (✉)
Department of Pediatrics and Division of Emergency Medicine, Louisiana State University Health Science Center, New Orleans, LA, USA

C. M. Zeretzke-Bien
Division of Pediatric Emergency Medicine, University of Florida, Gainesville, FL, USA
e-mail: Zeretzke@ufl.edu

© The Author(s), under exclusive license to Springer Nature
Switzerland AG 2023
C. M. Zeretzke-Bien, T. B. Swan (eds.), *Quick Hits for Pediatric Emergency Medicine*, https://doi.org/10.1007/978-3-031-32650-9_21

- Polyuria, polydipsia
- Breath has "fruity" odor
- Weight loss
- Tachypnea with deep, labored respirations (Kussmaul breathing)

• *Work-Up*

- Always assess and address ABCs prior to initiating treatment, especially in obtunded patients or clinically deteriorating patients.
- Labs

    Fingerstick glucose
    Blood gas
    CMP
    HbA1C
    UA (assess for glucosuria and ketonuria)
    CBC
    Consider beta-hydroxybutyric acid
    Consider work-up for any contributing factor such as infection if suspected

- If new onset diabetes, add the following labs:

    Islet cell antibodies
    Insulin antibodies
    Anti-GAD antibodies
    Thyroid antibodies
    Thyroid function tests
    Celiac screen (tissue transglutaminase and total immunoglobulin)
    Zinc transporter 8 autoantibody
    Ia2 autoantibody

• *Initial Stabilization and Treatment*

- NS or LR bolus (10–20 mL/kg over 1 h)
- Replete K+ if <3.5 mEq/L prior to insulin administration.
- Bicarbonate NOT indicated for routine treatment of acidosis in DKA
- May consider bicarbonate administration with EXTREME CAUTION if pH <6.9 *AND* cardiac or respiratory decompensation (should be used only with consult from endocrine or intensive care).
- Volume replacement

    Total fluid deficit = [estimated % dehydration × weight (kg)] × 1000 mL

- See chart below to estimate % dehydration. For most patients with DKA, one may assume 7% dehydration.

  Rate of rehydration fluids:

  - Over the next 48 h = (Total Fluid Deficit – Initial bolus)/48 h + hourly maintenance fluid requirement
  - Some advocate for a set rate of 1.5–2 times maintenance

  – Closely monitor for altered mental status, particularly if pH <7.15

    Consider hypertonic saline for concerns for cerebral edema

- *Insulin Treatment*

  – Start insulin infusion at 0.05–0.1 units/kg/h
  – DO NOT bolus with insulin
  – Do not start the insulin prior to confirmation that potassium is ≥3.5 mEq/L

- *Triple Bag Therapy for Moderate– Severe DK*

  – First bag: insulin as above
  – Second bag: 0.9% NaCl + 20 mEq K acetate + 20 mEq KPhos
  – Third bag: D10 0.9% NaCl + 20 mEq K acetate + 20 mEq KPhos

Fluid therapy should run at a constant rate during treatment. Percentage of total fluid rate for each fluid combination determined by hourly blood glucose:

Composition of rehydration fluids		
Blood glucose	NS +20 KPhos +20 KAc (%)	D10 NS +20 KPhos +20 KAc (%)
>350 mg/dL	100	0
250–350 mg/dL	50	50
<250 mg/dL	0	100

Most DKA patients will be suffering from moderate to severe dehydration. Estimated degree of dehydration and associated symptoms:

Mild (<5% dehydration)	Moderate (5–7%)	Severe (≥10%)
Dry mucous membranes Tachycardia	Capillary refill >2 s Sunken eyes Reduced skin turgor Absent tears All mild symptoms	Weak or non-palpable peripheral pulses Hypotension Shock Oliguria All mild and moderate symptoms

Quick Hit DKA Pearls

1. PECARN's (pediatric emergency care applied research network) recent clinical trial regarding fluid resuscitation in pediatric DKA indicates aggressive IV fluid resuscitation is not associated with increased clinically apparent cerebral injury. Specifically, there was no difference between 10 and 20 mL/kg or with rate of infusion in incidence of cerebral edema.
2. Obtain blood glucose checks every hour once insulin infusion initiated.
3. If patient has insulin pump, it must be removed prior to initiating insulin.
4. Insulin infusion should not be stopped until the patient is no longer acidotic; the anion gap is closed; and the patient is able to tolerate PO.
5. Most common causes of DKA:

    (a) Poor or noncompliance with insulin
    (b) Acute illness
    (c) Undiagnosed type 1 diabetes

Chapter 22
Pediatric Metabolic Emergencies

Sadiqa A. I. Kendi and Carmen J. Martinez

Abstract Metabolic emergencies must be considered in a pediatric patient presenting with vomiting, lethargy, irritability, altered mental status, seizures, or shock. This chapter includes "Quick Hits" and a pathway for consideration of adrenal crisis versus inborn errors of metabolism (IEM). The metabolic emergency pearls are a must-know in pediatric emergency medicine.

Adrenal crisis is a life-threatening illness that can occur in patients with adrenal insufficiency when under physiological stress (illness, trauma, surgery). Management involves the rapid reestablishment of normal perfusion, correction of electrolyte abnormalities, and administration of glucocorticoids.

Inborn errors of metabolism (IEM) are a set of various genetic disorders involving enzymatic deficiencies. As a result, metabolic pathways involved in the breakdown of nutrients and clearance of metabolites are abnormal and result in a toxic accumulation of substrates.

S. A. I. Kendi
Department of Pediatrics, Division of Pediatric Emergency Medicine, Boston University
Chobanian and Avedisian School of Medicine, Boston Medical Center, Boston, MA, USA

C. J. Martinez (✉)
Department of Emergency Medicine, Division of Pediatric Emergency Medicine, University
of South Alabama, USA Health Children's and Women's Hospital, Mobile, AL, USA
e-mail: cmartinez@health.southalabama.edu

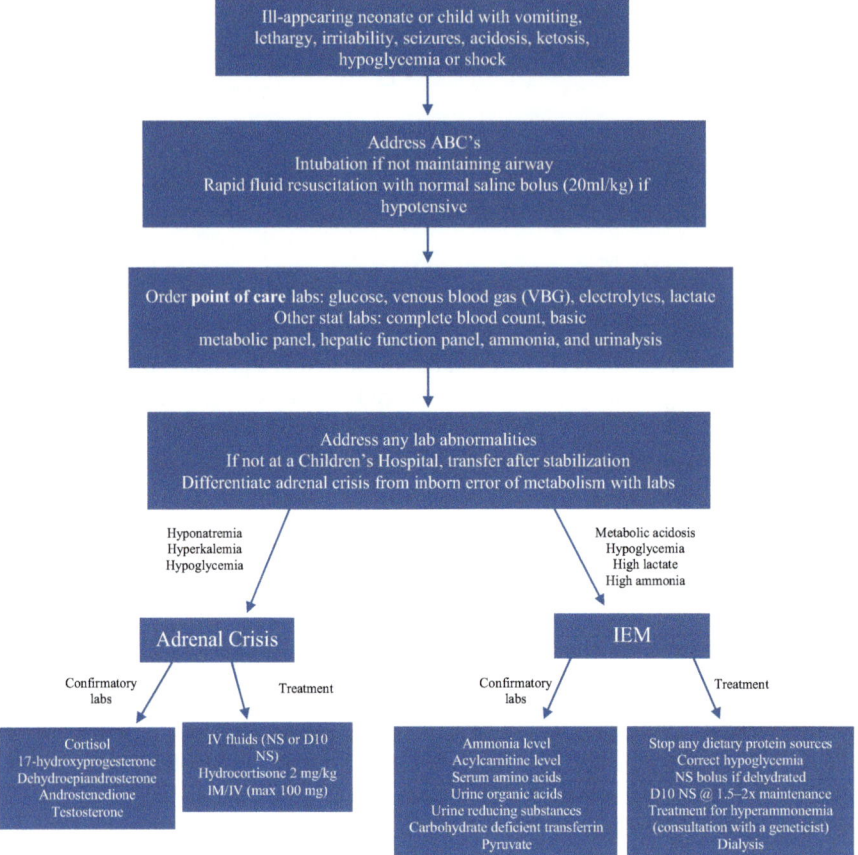

Interpretation of Serum Ammonia and ABG or VBG in Metabolic Diseases

ABG or VBG	Elevated serum ammonia	Normal serum ammonia
Metabolic acidosis	Fatty acid oxidation defects Methylmalonic acidemia Propionic acidemia	Some organic acidemias Maple syrup urine disease
Normal pH	Urea cycle defect	Galactosemia Aminoacidopathy Non-ketotic hyperglycinemia

Quick Hits Pediatric Metabolic Emergency Pearls

1. Consider metabolic emergencies in any ill-appearing child, especially an ill-appearing neonate.
2. Inborn errors of metabolism typically present in the neonatal period; however, they may present at ANY AGE so they must remain on your differential diagnosis at all times!
3. Remember a child with a history of chronic steroid use who is ill may present with a secondary adrenal crisis.
4. Look for electrolyte abnormalities, acidosis, and hypoglycemia.
5. Think dextrose (D10) fluids and give hydrocortisone early if inborn error of metabolism or adrenal crisis diagnosis is suspected.

Chapter 23
Pediatric Point-of-Care Ultrasound (POCUS)

Matthew Henry and Sakina H. Sojar

Abstract Recent focus has demonstrated point-of-care ultrasound (POCUS) to be an invaluable tool in the pediatric acute care setting. Interpretation can be performed in real time at the bedside, expediting appropriate care without delay or removal of the patient from the emergency department. With regard to considerations specific to the pediatric population, it serves as the diagnostic modality of choice for certain pathologies and may reduce the need for higher-risk studies (e.g. radiation from CT), reduce healthcare costs, shorten ED length-of-stay, and improve first pass success rates for various procedural applications.

M. Henry
Department of Pediatrics, University of Florida College of Medicine, UF Health Shands Children's Hospital, Gainesville, FL, USA
e-mail: mhenry2@ufl.edu

S. H. Sojar (✉)
Department of Emergency Medicine, Division of Pediatric Emergency Medicine, Warren Alpert Medical School of Brown University, Providence, RI, USA
e-mail: sakina.sojar@brownphysicians.org

Utility of Point-of-Care Ultrasound (POCUS) in Pediatric Emergency Medicine

Exam	Indication	Probe type	Key points
E-FAST	Rapid assessment for presence of free fluid or intervenable internal injuries after trauma, *especially in hypotensive patients*	Curvilinear or phased array	For intra-abdominal free fluid: RUQ view (liver caudal edge/tip) is most sensitive in older children; suprapubic most sensitive in prepubertal children. Overall less sensitive than in adults Pneumothorax: more sensitive than CXR in supine trauma patient
Cardiac	Assess gross function, presence of pericardial effusion, presence of right ventricular strain, etiology of shock to guide fluid resuscitation	Phased array	Subxiphoid view most sensitive for pericardial effusion Right ventricular strain best identified in short-axis view Comprehensive echocardiography preferred for suspected congenital heart lesions
Lung	Assess for pleural effusion, presence of b-lines (consolidation vs. edema), pneumonia, pneumothorax; guidance of chest tube placement	Linear	All high yield findings arise from the pleural line 1-2 B-lines in an area of lung can be normal, but more than 3 B-lines in a rib space is pathologic Pneumothorax: look for absent lung sliding of the pleural lines or "barcode sign" in M-mode Pneumonia: *dynamic air bronchograms* in the setting of consolation ("lung hepatization") most sensitive/specific; may have adjacent B-lines. Static bronchograms represent atelectasis vs infiltrate Lack of bronchograms with small subpleural consolidation and/or multiple/congruent B-lines suggests viral pathologies (bronchiolitis, etc.)
OB	Confirm intrauterine pregnancy, check fetal HR, assess for ovarian torsion with Doppler studies	Curvilinear or endocavitary	Fetal HR can be measured using M-mode Free fluid in Morrison's pouch raises concern for ectopic pregnancy
Renal/bladder	Measure bladder volume, assess for hydronephrosis, assess for ureteral obstruction	Curvilinear or phased array	Serial POCUS to *assess bladder fullness* prior to female pelvic ultrasound or neonatal urine catheterization reduces time to completion and improves first-try success

Exam	Indication	Probe type	Key points
Skin/soft tissue	Concern for cellulitis vs. abscess vs. foreign body	Linear	Cellulitis is diagnosed with the presence of "cobblestoning" Abscess may be diagnosed with spherical or oblong hypoechoic area with debris Squish sign for pus Consider adding color to assess for hyperemia suggestive of inflammation and to ensure no surrounding vessels prior to I+D procedure
Appendicitis	Right lower quadrant pain, anorexia, vomiting, fever	Linear (can consider curvilinear in larger patients)	Initial imaging modality of choice in pediatric patients over CT (no radiation, cheaper) Placing probe over most painful site may improve visualization success Diameter >6 mm
Intussusception	Toddler with intermittent bouts of abdominal pain; *young infant with isolated lethargy*	Linear	Small bowel-small bowel intussusceptions are typically smaller than ileocolic (<2 cm vs ≥2.5 cm) and may self-resolve Most commonly identified on the right side
Pyloric stenosis	Non-bilious projectile vomiting after every feed in 4–6 week old infant	Linear	If negative, cannot exclude other diagnoses (midgut volvulus vs malrotation) Anterior pyloric muscle wall thickness >3mm or channel length >14mm is abnormal
IV placement	Difficult IV access requiring real time visualization	Linear	Can improve first time success rate, catheter survival time, and time to completion Saphenous and antecubital veins may be best in children <3 years Shorter catheters (rather than US needles) preferred for infants
Nerve block	Anesthesia for procedure, minimizing need for procedural sedation	Linear	Use of POCUS may reduce risk of local anesthetic toxicity, adjacent structural damage, and overall success rates Nerves follow vascular bundles and travel within muscular fascial planes High yield locations: – Foot FB removal: posterior tibial n – Finger/hand reductions: ulnar/radial/median n – Extremity fractures: e.g. femoral n. or fascia iliaca for femur fracture

Pediatric-Specific Indications

Intussusception

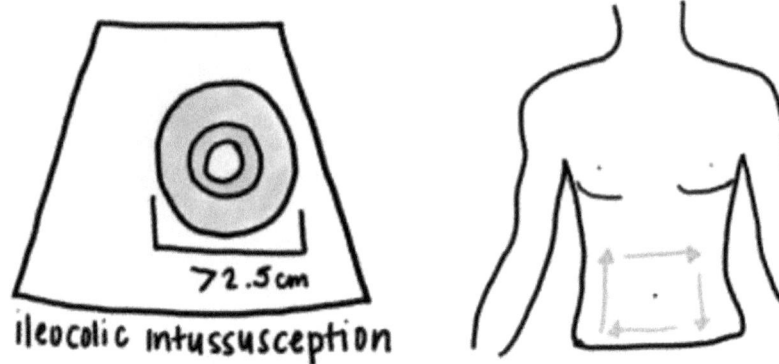

ileocolic intussusception

Diagnostic Findings: "Target sign" in short axis (pictured above), or "crescent in a doughnut sign" in transverse orientation

   Measurement: >2.5 cm usually consistent with ileo-colic intussusception (vs. ileo-ileo/small bowel, <2 cm)

   Technique:

1. Linear probe first placed in transverse orientation in RLQ to look for cecum.
2. Follow intestine superiorly to liver.
3. Rotate probe 90° clockwise and follow transverse colon in longitudinal orientation to LUQ.
4. Return to transverse orientation and follow the bowel to LLQ.
5. Screen the remainder of the bowel by sweeping back-and-forth across the full abdomen.

Appendicitis

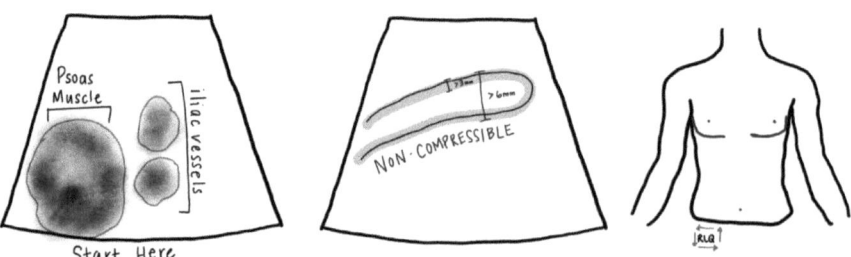

Diagnostic Findings: Non-compressible, non-peristalsing blind-ending tubular structure arising from the cecum, "ring of fire" on doppler suggestive of peri-appendiceal edema, and/or presence of appendicolith/fecalith

Measurement: diameter >6 mm

Technique:

1. Linear probe placed at McBurney's point (1/3 distance from anterior superior iliac spine to umbilicus) or point of maximum tenderness in RLQ.
2. If unsuccessful, locate the psoas muscle and iliac vessels, starting just inferior to the iliac crest and move up towards the head.
3. May require graded compression to move excess bowel gas which can obstruct your view.
4. It is noteworthy to offer patient analgesia prior to performing this exam, as compression can be extremely painful in the setting of appendicitis.

Pyloric Stenosis

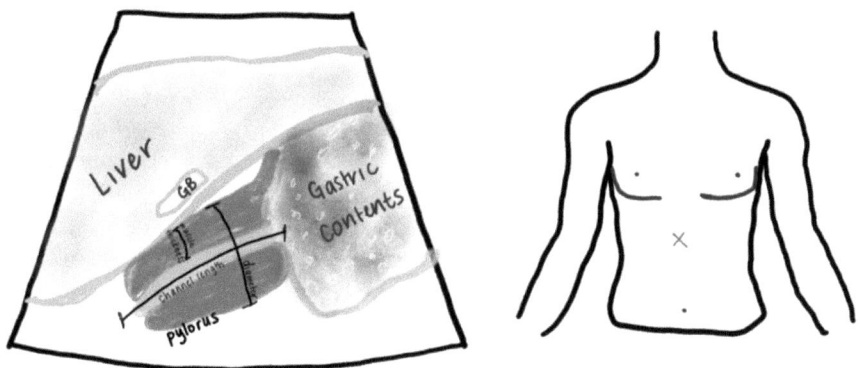

Diagnostic Finding: Thickened wall of the pylorus, elongated pyloric channel, stomach contents do not pass through pylorus.

Measurements >3 mm anterior wall thickness, or channel length >14 mm (think Pi, "3.14").

Technique:

1. Feeding the infant will allow for better visualization of stomach/pylorus.
2. Place infant in right lateral decubitus, ideally while feeding in parent's lap.
3. Use linear probe in transverse orientation in the subxiphoid area to assess epigastrium just right of midline.
4. As stomach fills, identify the antrum of the stomach and follow the anterior gastric wall to the pylorus.
5. Regardless of measurements, if fluid is seen passing through the pylorus into the duodenum, the study is negative.

Peripheral IV Placement

Helpful Tips:

Veins with the highest success/IV longevity are >3 mm diameter and between 0.5 and 1 cm in depth, without bifurcations and straight.

Be aware of surrounding anatomy (arteries, nerves, etc.) and needed catheter length depending on depth.

Providers generally perform this procedure in the transverse/out of plane view where it is important to know the location of your needle tip at all times.

Technique (Out of Plane):

1. Insert the needle at a 45-degree angle and locate the tip with your probe.
2. Advance probe until tip is no longer visible; advance needle until tip again visualized adjusting the catheter angle to guide tip towards vessel.
3. Alternate advancing probe and needle until the tip just touches the vessel lumen, then decrease catheter angle and advance.

Quick Hits Pediatric POCUS Pearls:

1. Pediatric POCUS has a wide variety of applications including the E-FAST exam, and evaluation for appendicitis, pyloric stenosis, intussusception. and IV placement.
2. Utilization of Pediatric POCUS can reduce radiation exposure to children.
3. Correct probe selection is vital to the exam type you are conducting!

References

1. Hopkins A, Doniger SJ. Point-of-care ultrasound for the pediatric hospitalist's practice. Hosp Pediatr. 2019;9(9):707–18. https://doi.org/10.1542/hpeds.2018-0118. Epub 2019 Aug 12. PMID: 31405888.
2. Lin-Martore M, Kornblith AE. Diagnostic applications of point-of-care ultrasound in pediatric emergency medicine. Emerg Med Clin North Am. 2021;39(3):509–27. https://doi.org/10.1016/j.emc.2021.04.005. PMID: 34215400.
3. Persson JN, Kim JS, Good RJ. Diagnostic utility of point-of-care ultrasound in the pediatric cardiac intensive care unit. Curr Treat Options Pediatr. 2022;8(3):151–73. https://doi.org/10.1007/s40746-022-00250-1. Epub 2022 Jul 8. PMID: 36277259; PMCID: PMC9264295.
4. Singh Y, Tissot C, Fraga MV, Yousef N, Cortes RG, Lopez J, Sanchez-de-Toledo J, Brierley J, Colunga JM, Raffaj D, Da Cruz E, Durand P, Kenderessy P, Lang HJ, Nishisaki A, Kneyber MC, Tissieres P, Conlon TW, De Luca D. International evidence-based guidelines on Point of Care Ultrasound (POCUS) for critically ill neonates and children issued by the POCUS Working Group of the European Society of Paediatric and Neonatal Intensive Care (ESPNIC). Crit Care. 2020;24(1):65. https://doi.org/10.1186/s13054-020-2787-9. PMID: 32093763; PMCID: PMC7041196.

Chapter 24
Pediatric Obstetric, Gynecologic, and Urologic Emergencies

Juan Carlos Gonzalez and Tricia B. Swan

Abstract In the pediatric emergency room, obstetrical and urological emergencies can be challenging and require prompt attention. Management of these emergencies often involves a multidisciplinary approach, with close collaboration between emergency physicians, obstetricians, and urologists. This Quick Hits chapter will help you recognize and treat acute genitourinary emergencies in children. Timely and accurate diagnosis, along with appropriate intervention and consultation, can help ensure optimal outcomes for these vulnerable patients. Additionally, careful consideration should be given to the unique needs of pediatric patients, including their developmental stage and emotional state, to minimize stress and maximize comfort during evaluation and treatment.

Vaginitis

	Normal flora	Bacterial vaginosis	Vulvovaginal candidiasis	Trichomoniasis
pH	<4.5	>4.5	<4.5	Normal or >4.5
Microscopy findings	Lactobacillus present with some WBCs	Clue cells	Hyphae may be seen	Trichomonads may be seen with an abundant WBC
Whiff test (KOH test)	Not applicable	Positive	Negative	Variable
Treatment	None	Metronidazole 500 mg BID × 7 days	Fluconazole 150 mg PO × 1 dose	Metronidazole 500 mg BID × 7 days

J. C. Gonzalez (✉)
Department of Emergency Medicine, Division of Pediatric Emergency Medicine, University of Florida College of Medicine, UF Health Shands Children's Hospital, Gainesville, FL, USA
e-mail: Juan.gonzalez@ufl.edu

T. B. Swan
Division of Pediatric Emergency Medicine, University of Florida, Gainesville, FL, USA
e-mail: tfalgiani@ufl.edu

© The Author(s), under exclusive license to Springer Nature Switzerland AG 2023
C. M. Zeretzke-Bien, T. B. Swan (eds.), *Quick Hits for Pediatric Emergency Medicine*, https://doi.org/10.1007/978-3-031-32650-9_24

Pelvic Inflammatory Disease

Minimum Criteria to Diagnosis

- Sexually active patient with pelvic or lower abdominal pain, with no other causes identified and one of the following:

  - Cervical motion tenderness *OR*
  - Uterine tenderness *OR*
  - Adnexal tenderness

- The following findings enhance the specificity of the minimum criteria:

  - Oral temperature >101 F
  - Abnormal cervical or vaginal discharge
  - Abundant numbers of WBC on microscopy
  - ESR >15 mm/h or elevated CRP
  - Documented gonococcal or chlamydial cervical infection

- Treatment for Pelvic Inflammatory Disease includes the following:

  - 1 g of ceftriaxone PLUS
  - Doxycycline 100 mg PO BID × 14 days PLUS
  - Metronidazole 500 mg PO BID × 14 days

Adnexal (Ovarian) Torsion

The most common clinical symptom of adnexal torsion is sudden onset of abdominal pain that is intermittent, non-radiating and is frequently associated with nausea and vomiting. It is important to recognize that these symptoms can be vague and can be caused by many other etiologies; therefore, adnexal torsion should ALWAYS be on the differential diagnosis for female patients with abdominal pain. Plan for these patients include:

- Urinalysis and urine culture
- Urine pregnancy test
- Pelvic US with Doppler to assess the adnexa

  - Most common finding on US in children with ovarian torsion is an enlarged ovary.
  - Due to the dual blood supply of the ovary, Doppler findings can be inconsistent; therefore, demonstration of blood flow should **NOT** definitely rule out torsion.

If examination or history is concerning for or torsion of the adnexa is suspected, patients should be placed NPO with a consultation to gynecology or surgery for diagnostic and therapeutic laparoscopy.

Abnormal Uterine Bleeding

Uterine bleeding is considered abnormal if:

- There is bleeding or spotting between periods.
- Menstrual cycles that are longer than 35 days or shorter than 21 days.
- Irregular cycles in which the length varies by more than 7 days.
- Not having a period for 3–6 months.
- Heavy bleeding during the period

    - Bleeding that lasts more than 7 days.
    - Bleeding that soaks though one or more pads/tampons every hour.

	Mild AUB	Moderate AUB	Severe AUB
Hemoglobin level	>12.0 g/dL	10–12 g/dL	<10 g/dL
Iron supplementation	Can consider	Will require 65 mg/day	Will require 65 mg/day
Disposition	Can follow up in the outpatient setting with their PCP	Can follow up in the outpatient setting with their PCP and other specialists including OB/GYN. Will require ethinyl estradiol 0.03 mg/norgestrel 0.3 mg OCP q6 hours until bleeding stops	May require admission depending on hemodynamic stability If bleeding is severe and poorly controlled, Premarin 35 mgIV q4 hours × 3 doses Otherwise ethinylestradiol 0.05 mg/norgestrel 0.5 mg OCP q6 hours until bleeding stops

Contraindications to estrogen containing medications:

- History of migraine with aura
- History of DVT
- Inherited prothrombotic disorders
- SLE with positive or unknown antiphospholipid antibodies
- Hypertension

- Heart or liver conditions
- Postpartum <21 days
- Current diagnosis of breast cancer
- History of solid organ transplant

Pregnancy

Recent research has shown approximately 50% of high school students have been sexually active. Of those who are sexually active, 60% report condom use and 20% report birth control. Pediatric ER visits for pregnancy account for less than 1% of all visits. It is important to consider performing a pregnancy test in any peri- or post-menarche female.

- Once a diagnosis of pregnancy has been established, goals in the emergency department include:

  - Disclose the diagnosis of pregnancy to ONLY the patient and determine patient safety and willingness to share the diagnosis with others. Being aware of local and state laws regarding a sexually related diagnosis is critical to emergency department providers.
  - Assessing for ectopic versus intrauterine pregnancy.
  - Dating the pregnancy.
  - Recognizing symptoms that require referral to OBGYN.
  - Identifying and treating potential nonsurgical complications.
  - Determination if the pregnancy resulted from sexual abuse or assault.
  - Providing counseling and securing appropriate and timely follow-up.

    It is best to have follow-up scheduled in 2–3 days with either PCP, adolescent medicine, or OBGYN.

- Evaluation should include quantitative serum B-hCG levels, serum progesterone levels, and pelvic ultrasound.

  - In the first four weeks of pregnancy B-hCG levels should double every 48–72 h.
  - Levels that do not rise or rise more slowly than expected are indicative of an abnormal pregnancy (usually ectopic or a pregnancy that is destined to spontaneously abort) (Fig. 24.1).
  - A progesterone level greater than 25 ng/dL is seen in 95% of normal pregnancies; a level <5 ng/dL suggests an abnormal pregnancy.

Classifications of Spontaneous Abortions

Missed

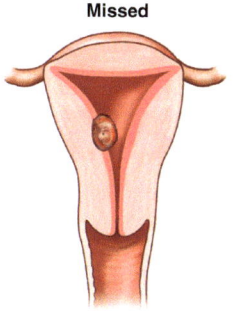

- No vaginal bleeding
- Closed cervical os
- No fetal cardiac activity or empty sac

Threatened

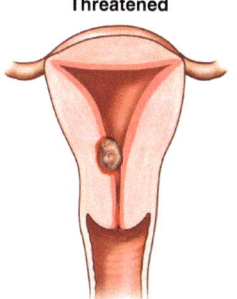

- Vaginal bleeding and cramping
- Cervix closed and soft
- Fetal cardiac activity

Inevitable

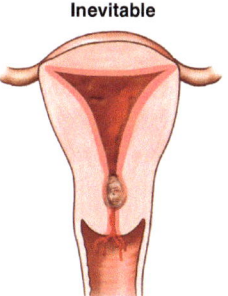

- Vaginal bleeding and cramping
- Rupture of membranes
- Dilated cervical os
- Products of conception may be seen or felt at or above cervical os

Incomplete

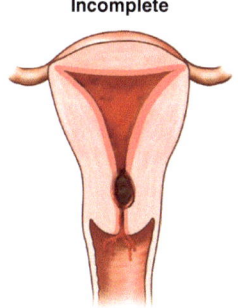

- Vaginal bleeding and cramping
- Dilated cervical os
- Some products of conception expelled

Complete

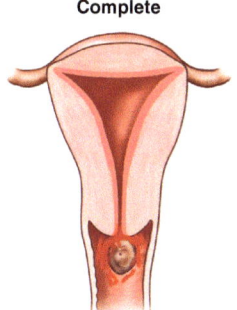

- Vaginal bleeding
- Closed cervical os
- Products of conception completely expelled

Fig. 24.1 Classifications of spontaneous abortions

Ectopic Pregnancy

- Leading cause of maternal mortality in the USA during the first half of pregnancy.
- Prevalence of ectopic pregnancy presenting to emergency departments ranges from 5 to 15%.
- Risk factors include prior ectopic pregnancy, tubal abnormalities, prior upper genital tract infection, and assisted reproduction.

- Patients can present with a wide variety of symptoms including vaginal bleeding, crampy lower abdominal pain, or examination suggestive of an acute abdomen with or without shock.
- For patients diagnosed with ectopic pregnancy, conservative medical management may be appropriate in patients who are:
  - Hemodynamically stable
  - Have no evidence of bleeding
  - Have a hemoglobin level > 8 g/dL
  - A gestational sac <4 cm
  - Are immunocompetent
  - Do not have a bleeding diathesis, live, or renal disease.
  - Proper close follow-up with OB/GYN can be ensured.

- If a patient presents with an acutely ruptured ectopic pregnancy, they need immediate OBGYN or pediatric surgery consultation and fluid resuscitation.

Urological Emergencies

Urethral Prolapse

- Peak age for urethral prolapse in prepubertal children is between 5 and 8 years old.
- Presents as a doughnut shaped protrusion from the vulva and happen spontaneously.
- Vaginal bleeding or spotting is the chief complaint in 90% of children with urethral prolapse.
- If dark red or necrotic tissue is present, urgent surgical consultation is required for reduction of the prolapsed tissue (Fig. 24.2a, b).
- If necrotic tissue is not present, management includes warm compresses or sitz baths with a 2-week course of topical estrogen.

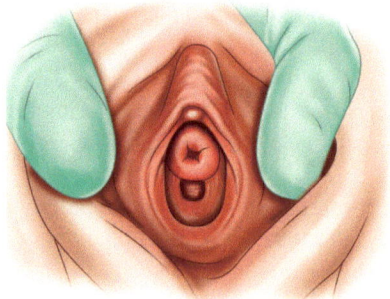

Fig. 24.2 Urethral prolapse

Phimosis and Paraphimosis

- Phimosis

  - Defined as the inability to retract the foreskin. The incidence of fully retract-able foreskin increases with age as the rate of phimosis decreases.
  - Physiologic: Seen in almost all newborn males due to normal development of congenital adhesions between foreskin and glans.
  - Pathologic: Foreskin that is truly nonretractable secondary to distal scarring of the prepuce.
  - In children over 2 years of age, the foreskin should be able to be retracted to the point where the urethral meatus is visible.
  - In the newborn, the foreskin requires no particular care other than what is provided to the rest of the body. Avoid forcible retraction because tearing may cause bleeding and fibrosis.
  - Phimosis does not require emergent treatment.
  - Treatment of phimosis is application of 0.05% betamethasone cream twice a day for 6 weeks.

- Paraphimosis

  - Refers to retracted foreskin in an uncircumcised or partially circumcised male that cannot be returned to a normal position.
  - Patient will present with severe penile pain with swelling of the glans penis and distal foreskin due to the constricting band of tissue present at the coronal sulcus.
  - Treatment is emergent and includes pain control, manual reduction, or a dorsal slit reduction (with a consult to urology if possible).
  - Manual reduction may be accomplished by applying ice and steady manual compression on the swollen foreskin ring (Fig. 24.3).

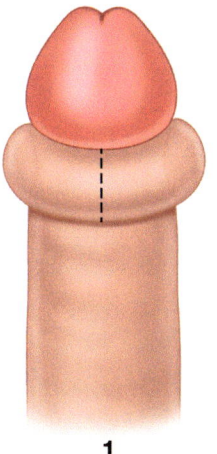
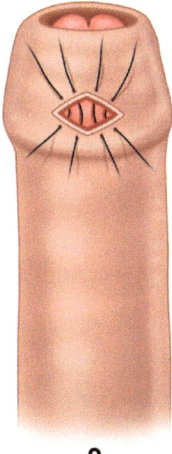
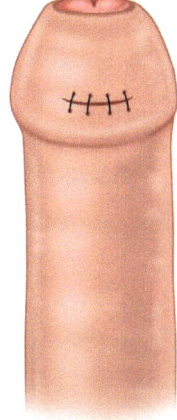

1   **2**   **3**

Fig. 24.3 Dorsal slit reduction

– Doral slit reduction

> Incision is made along the dorsal skin longitudinally for 1–2 cm over the constriction. This will allow edema to flow past the ring and decrease glans edema so that the foreskin can be returned to a normal position.
> After reduction, the patient should not retract the foreskin for approximately 1 week.

Balanitis and Balanoposthitis

- Balanitis is pain and inflammation of the glans of the penis.
- Balanoposthitis is pain and inflammation of both the glans and foreskin.
- Patient may have a preceding history of bite or small punctate lesion to the area.
- Treatment is aimed at cause of inflammation or infection and may include warm soaks, topical antifungal medication if candidiasis is suspected or treatment with a first generation cephalosporin (or clindamycin if allergic) if cellulitis is suspected.

Meatal Stenosis

- Seen exclusively in circumcised males and usually follows an inflammatory reaction around the meatus. Usually occurs from the meatus rubbing against a wet diaper. Significant meatal stenosis causes spraying of the urinary stream or more commonly dorsal deflection of the stream.

Priapism

- Prolonged, painful penile erection unaccompanied by sexual stimulation. Generally lasting longer than 4 h.
- May be caused by trauma or leukemic infiltration but most often seen in males with sickle cell disease.

- Labs include:
  - Urinalysis and urine culture, CBC, LFTs, LDH, CRP, and coagulation studies.
- Treatment includes hydration, oxygen, and analgesia followed by irrigation of the corporal bodies with saline with phenylephrine 250–500 µg/cc in conjunction with urgent consultation with a urologist.

Testicular Torsion

- Torsion accounts for 10–15% of acute scrotal pain.
- Two peaks, once in the newborn period and the other around puberty.
- Typically presents with acute, severe pain with nausea and vomiting and pain is not relieved by any position.
- In newborns, may present as sudden enlargement and redness of the hemiscrotum.
- May present as abdominal pain alone (any boy with abdominal pain must undergo a testicular exam).
- The torsed testis may have a horizontal lie and may lie higher in the scrotum than the contralateral testis, with absent cremasteric reflex on the affected side.
- Color Doppler US can help with evaluation of testis and can help show decreased or absent arterial blood flow. If torsion is on the differential, consult urological surgery immediately for exploration and repair of the testis! DO NOT DELAY! (Fig. 24.4)
- Treatment of torsion is surgical exploration, detorsion, and fixation of the bilateral testis.
- Use the TWIST score if testicular torsion is a concern.

Nausea or vomiting	1 point
Testicular swelling	2 points
Hard testis on palpation	2 points
High riding testis	1 point
Absent cremasteric reflex	1 point

A score of greater than or equal to 5 is indicative of testicular torsion with a specificity of 100% and a PPV of 100%. A score of <2 excludes testicular torsion with a sensitivity of 100% and a NPV of 100%

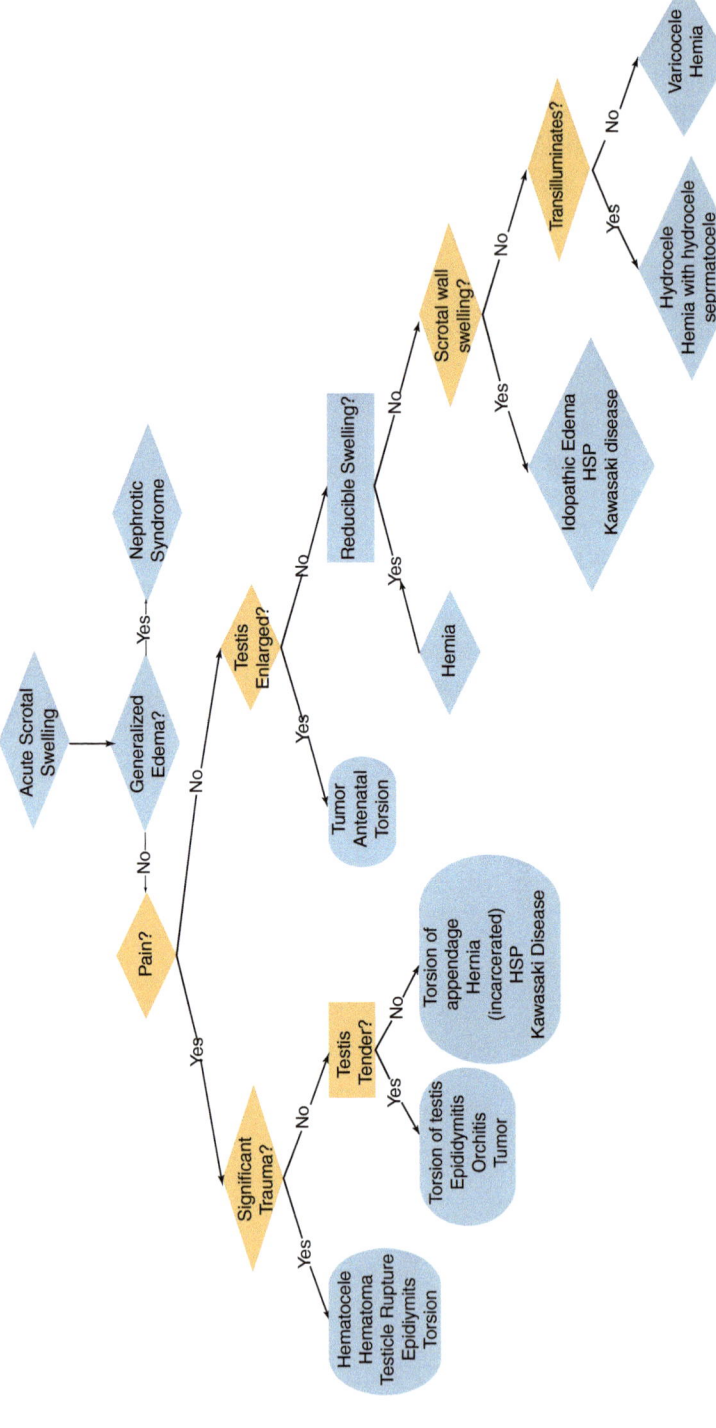

Fig. 24.4 Acute scrotal swelling pathway

Epididymitis

- Can present very similarly to testicular torsion.
- Typically, not associated with nausea or vomiting
- The scrotum may be enlarged and erythematous.
- In prepubertal boys this is idiopathic or may be due to chemical irritation. In post-pubertal boys, they may be secondary to an STI including gonorrhoeae or chlamydia.

  – Treatment includes NSAIDS, ice, and scrotal support. If urine culture is positive, they should be treated empirically with antibiotics.

Renal Colic/Nephrolithiasis

- The primary goal in the acute setting is diagnosing obstruction and providing pain control, nausea control, hydration, and education.
- Emergent if renal stone is associated with fevers (infected stone or sepsis) or if there is an obstructing stone in patient with solitary kidney.
- Patients presenting with flank pain with or without the presence of hematuria should be evaluated for a kidney stone with US imaging as the first line.
- Management includes hydration and pain control with narcotics or NSAIDS if there is no evidence of renal dysfunction.
- If there is a suspected stone and the ultrasound is abnormal and does not show the stone, a noncontract CT scan can be obtained.
- Treatment

  – If non-obstructing and not infected, medical expulsion therapy alone, including pain medication, and tamsulosin.
  – If the stone is obstructive, then surgical decompression is required.

Acute Urinary Retention

- May be caused by numerous etiologies. Severe constipation, bladder outlet obstruction from posterior urethral valves or obstructing ureteroceles, drugs, post-operative states, or toxins must be considered.
- For children with voluntary retention, gentile massage of the lower abdomen with a soak in a warm tub leads to the spontaneous evacuation of the bladder.
- If unable to void, drainage with bladder catheter can be done.
- If the child has had a history of bladder augmentation or unable to pass a catheter, the bladder can be drained with a transabdominal needle.

How to Do a Suprapubic Aspiration of a bladder

- Absolute contraindications
  - Skin or soft tissue infection of the abdominal wall over the bladder
- Relative contraindications
  - Empty bladder
  - Major GU abnormalities
  - Bleeding disorder
  - Massive hepatosplenomegaly
  - Previous abdominal surgery
- Equipment
  - Sterile drapes and gloves
  - Antiseptic solution
  - Lidocaine, 25-gauge needle, and a 5 mL syringe
  - A 5 mL syringe, 22-guage 1.5 inch needle for aspiration
  - Sterile cup for urine specimen
- Procedure
  - Locate the bladder by the use of point-of-care ultrasound. Cover the ultrasound probe with a sterile cover and place the probe on the abdominal wall just inferior to the planned needle insertion site.
  - Locate the point of entry, which is 1–2 cm cephalad to the superior edge of the symphysis pubis in the midline.
  - Clean the area from the pubic symphysis to the umbilicus with antiseptic solution.
  - Inject local anesthetic subcutaneously and into the dermis at the planned site.
  - Insert a 22-gauge needle attached to a 5 mL syringe into the entry site perpendicular to the abdominal wall.
  - With the ultrasound, follow the needle as it advances through the anterior abdominal wall and into the bladder. When the needle is in the bladder, aspirate the urine.
  - After collecting adequate urine, withdraw the syringe and needle, place a bandage over the puncture site.

Quick Hits Pediatric Obstetric, Gynecologic, and Urologic Emergencies Pearls

1. A complete genitourinary examination is critical for all patients who present with abdominal pain.
2. With any GU complaint or emergency ensure the patient can urinate prior to discharging them home.
3. Patients with abnormal uterine bleeding must be immediately assessed for hemodynamic stability.
4. Patient confidentiality regarding sexually related diagnoses must be maintained in accordance with local and state law.
5. The diagnosis of adnexal (ovarian) torsion can be extremely difficult to make due to lack of specific and sensitive history and physical examination findings, therefore must always be on your differential for female abdominal pain.
6. Testicular torsion in males may present as abdominal pain alone: you MUST do a testicular examination on any male presenting with abdominal pain!

Chapter 25
Approach to Vulnerable Populations

Cristina M. Zeretzke-Bien

Abstract Trauma informed care, tonic immobility, fight, flight, freeze, labor trafficking, human trafficking, reporting hotline, bruises, bites, irritability, mandated reporter, suspicious fracture.

A Word on Vulnerable Populations
Trauma Informed Care

We should all be aware of the Neurobiology of Trauma.

- High stress and fear impair our prefrontal cortex so one "cannot think straight."
- We cannot focus our attention, draw on reason or past experience, cannot think it through or inhibit our impulses.
- Results in a FIGHT FLIIGHT FREEZE state

    - Self-protection habits kick in

        being polite to dominant/aggressive people

    - Disassociation is common

        blanked out/spaced out/fog/dream

C. M. Zeretzke-Bien (✉)
Division of Pediatric Emergency Medicine, University of Florida, Gainesville, FL, USA
e-mail: Zeretzke@ufl.edu

C. M. Zeretzke-Bien, T. B. Swan (eds.), *Quick Hits for Pediatric Emergency Medicine*, https://doi.org/10.1007/978-3-031-32650-9_25

– Tonic immobility

> frozen state—cannot move or speak can last seconds to hours

– As a result of the cascade of hormonal and chemical changes from trauma patients do not lay down memory in a sequential pattern.

> Comes across in "Bits and pieces" of memory

Human Trafficking/Labor Trafficking

- **What is Human Trafficking?** The act of coercion, fraud, or forcing a person into leaving their home to work for little or no payment.
- **What is Labor Trafficking?** The recruitment, harboring, transportation, provision, or obtaining of a person for labor or services through force, coercion, or fraud.

  – *Child victims often present with complaints related to their experience trafficking*
  – These include:

  > work-related injuries
  > exposure to toxins
  > bruises and scars
  > exhaustion
  > malnutrition (See Fig. 25.1)

To harbor safe interactions one needs to remember to:

- Keep the survivor on the forefront of our interactions—*Victim Centered*
- Safe space
- Traumas create *triggers* (sights, sounds, emotions)
- Send an *authentic* message
- Realizes the widespread impact of trauma
- Responds by integrations of knowledge
- Seeks to resist re-traumatization

Red Flags to Identify Human Trafficking victims:

Physical Exam
- *General Appearance*: Appears malnourished, limping /pain
- *Skin:* Trauma, scars, rashes, sunburn, track marks, branding
- *Gyn/GU:* STI, trauma, foreign bodies, unknown pregnancy

Other Signs
- Lack of control
- Minor not in school
- Does not speak English
- Alcohol/drugs
- Trauma
- Unfamiliar with surroundings

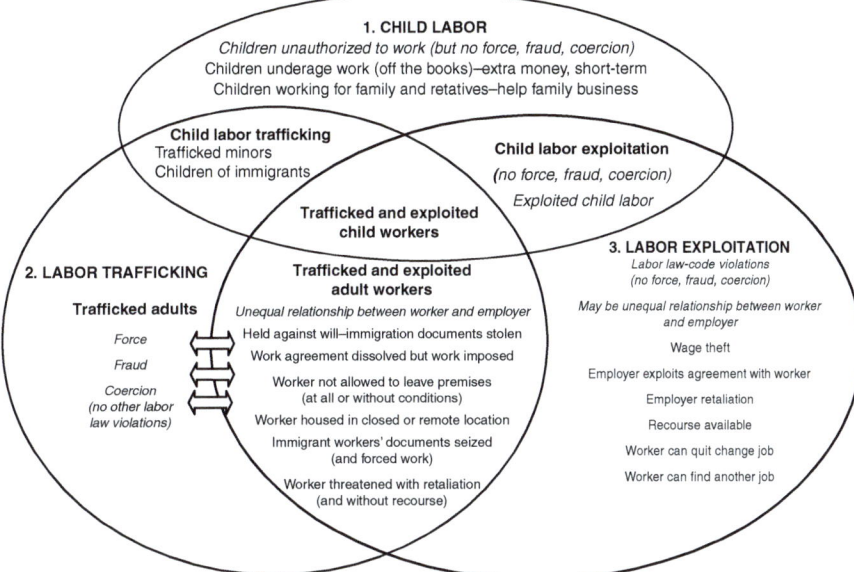

Fig. 25.1   Child labour

68% of Human Trafficking Victims access Healthcare While Being Trafficked!

Every hospital or institution should have a protocol to report suspected victims
   National Reporting hotline: 1-888-373-7888

Child Abuse:

Means:

1. Intentional infliction of physical or mental injury upon a child
2. An intentional act that could reasonably be expected to result in physical or mental injury to a child.
3. Active encouragement of any person to commit an act that results or could reasonably be expected to result in physical or mental injury to a child.

Recognizing Child Abuse

Pay Attention to the Following

History
  Physical Examination
  Lab Studies

- The history does not explain the injury found.
- Multiple injuries of various types or ages
- Delay in seeing medical attention for an injury which is obviously serious.
- No history offered to explain an injury which is serious or typical of abuse.

Types of Discrepancies Between History and Injury

- History changes over time or different caretakers give different stories.
- Child is developmentally incapable of having acted as described.
- Child would not reasonably be expected to have acted as described.
- Serious injury blamed on another child.

Rules to Follow

1. Those that do not Cruise Rarely Bruise!
2. Follow the following TEN-4-FACES bruising rule
   TEN 4-FACES Bruising Rule
   Any bruise found in any of the following locations should trigger the possibility of pediatric physical abuse.
   Torso
   Ears
   Neck
   Any bruise in a child younger than 4 months old
   FACES
   Frenulum
   Angle of the Jaw
   Cheek
   Eyelid
   Subconjunctival Hemorrhage
3. Be AWARE of patterned bruises

   (a) Linear bruises to buttocks
   (b) Linear bruising to the pinna
   (c) Retinal bleeding
   (d) Handprints or oval marks

    (e) Belt marks

    (f) Loop Marks

    (g) Ligature marks, circumferential rope burns to the neck, wrists, ankles, or gag marks at the corners of the mouth

4. Too many bruises
5. Any fracture in a non-ambulatory child
6. Bonks (see Fig 25.2)
7. Bites—any human bites
8. Baby blues (irritability) (Fig. 25.3)

Question if Accidental

- How foreseeable and preventable was the accident?
- How do the caretaker's actions compare to the standard in the community?
- What is the overall level of concern about the child's welfare?
- What is the potential for the child to be injured again?

Pittsburgh Infant Brain Injury Score (PIBIS) for Abusive Head Trauma

The 5-point PIBIS

1. Abnormality on dermatologic examination (2 points),
2. Age ≥3.0 months (1 point),
3. Head circumference >85th percentile(1 point), and
4. Serum hemoglobin <11.2g/dL(1 point)

At a score of 2, the sensitivity and specificity for abnormal neuroimaging was 93.3% (95% confidence interval 89.0%–96.3%) and 53% (95% confidence interval 49.3%–57.1%), respectively.

Fig. 25.2 Pittsburgh infant brain injury score for abusive head trauma

Child Presenting with Injury		
Historical Indicators of Abuse	**The Physical Exam's 6 B's of Abuse**	**Injuries Suggestive of Abuse**
- Changing of evolving history - Injury not consistent with mechanism - Injury not consistent with development stage - Delay in seeking medical care - History of past injuries - Unexplained injuries/deaths in siblings	**Bruises:** Pre-mobile; TEN-4 (Torso, Ear, Neck) F.A.C.E.S (Frenulum, Angle of Jaw, Cheek, Eyelid, Subconjuctival); Patten; Too many **Breaks:** Needs a clear history. Unsual in very young. Ignore Toddler's Fracture **Bonks:** Worry if complex, bilateral, depressed, open, suture diathesis of occipital fracures **Bums:** Worry if bilateral, well demarcated, immersion pattern (glove & stocking) **Bites:** Unlikely to have innocent mechanism **Baby Blues:** Unexplained behavioral change	- Posterior rib fractures - Long bone fracrures if <6mo - Metaphyseal fractures - Scapular fractures - Vertebral fractures - Sternal fractures - Hand/foot fractures - Facial fractures - SDH - Unexplained TBI
Consider Reporting		

Fig. 25.3 Child presenting with injury

Fractures Highly Specific for Abuse

- Metaphyseal lesions
- Posterior rib fractures
- Scapular fractures
- Spinous process fractures
- Sternal fractures

Final Points

- We are advocates for children!
- Pay attention to clinical clues in history and the physical exam findings.
- Call for resources for families in need.
- We are mandated reporters.

   Do the right thing for the child, and help to prevent the future catastrophe!

Index

A

Abdominal pain
  classic electrolyte abnormalities in
      pyloric stenosis, 43
  complete physical exam, 43
  differential diagnosis for, 43
Abdominal trauma., 50
Abdominal X-ray, 41
Abnormal uterine bleeding, 175–176
Abort seizure, 109
Accessory respiratory muscles, 2
Acetaminophen, 130–132
Acidosis, 120
Activated charcoal, 129, 132
Acute/chronic renal failure, 116
Acute gastroenteritis, 43
Acute tubular necrosis, 117, 118
Acute urinary retention, 183
Acyclovir, 110
Adenoidal hypertrophy, 1
Adenosine, 25
Adenovirus, 9
Adnexal torsion, 174
Adrenal crisis, 163
Adrenal insufficiency, 116, 124
AEIOU TIPS, 86–87
Air enema, 42
Airways, 1
  before intubation
      cricoid cartilage, 1
      large occiput., 1
      large tongue, 1
      larynx, 1
      lung, physiology, 2
      mechanics, 2
      pediatric airway anatomy, 1
      vocal cords slant anteriorly, 1
  and cervical spine stabilization, 48
  management, 109
Airway adjuncts
  confirmation, 63
  depth, 63
  intraosseous access
      contraindications, 65
      distal femur, 65
      proximal tibia, 65
  sizing, 63
Airway inflammation, 6
Airway obstruction, 31
Airway protection, 56
Airway urgency, 7, 10
Albuterol, 6–8
Alcohol, 127
Alkalosis, 118
Altered mental status, 53, 115, 117, 121–123
  in children, 85–87
Alveoli, 2
Amiodarone, 25
Amoxicillin, 143–149, 156
Amoxicillin-clavulanate, 144, 145, 147–149
Ampicillin, 143–146, 148, 149, 156
Ankle Triplane, 79
Anterior interosseous nerve, 77
Antidotes, 128–131
Antiepileptic drugs (AEDs), 109
Antihistamines, 127
APGAR scores, 38
Apnea, 40
Apophysitis, 82–83
Appendicitis, 41, 43, 169–171

C. M. Zeretzke-Bien, T. B. Swan (eds.), *Quick Hits for Pediatric Emergency
Medicine*, https://doi.org/10.1007/978-3-031-32650-9